THE
COURTIN
CONCEPT

Six Keys to Great Skin
at Any Age

OLIVIER COURTIN-CLARINS, M.D.

Addicus Books
Omaha, Nebraska

An Addicus Nonfiction Book

ISBN# 978-1-886039-86-5

Cover and book design by Peri Poloni-Gabriel, www.knockoutbooks.com
Illustration by Jack Kusler

This book is not intended to serve as a substitute for a physician. Nor is it the author's intent to give medical advice contrary to that of an attending physician.

Library of Congress Cataloging-in-Publication Data

Courtin-Clarins, Olivier, 1954-
  The Courtin concept : six keys to great skin at any age / Olivier Courtin-Clarins.
     p. cm.
  Includes index.
  ISBN 978-1-886039-86-5 (alk. paper)
  1. Skin—Care and hygiene. 2. Beauty, Personal. 3. Cosmetics. I. Title.

RL87.C69 2007
646.7'2--dc22
                                   2007026442

 Addicus Books, Inc.
P.O. Box 45327
Omaha, Nebraska 68145
www.AddicusBooks.com

Printed in the United States of America

10   9   8   7   6   5   4   3   2   1

Contents

Acknowledgments

FIRST AND FOREMOST, I want to thank my father, Jacques Courtin, who has been my most important teacher when it comes to cosmetics and life. His deep insight and knowledge of human relationships have always been of great value to me.

I also thank my brother Christian for his constant encouragement when I started working for Clarins. All of my professors in medicine and surgery deserve recognition, as does Lionel de Benetti who has worked with me to build the international research network for Clarins.

I want to express appreciation to my two daughters, Prisca and Jenna, whose love has always been a true strength to me. During the writing of this book, the enthusiastic support of my nieces, Virginie and Claire, was also greatly appreciated.

A special thanks to all of my former patients; Harriet Tancerman, my English teacher; Shari Leslie Segall, who helped me with this book; Florence Grimault, my assistant; David Applefield, my publishing consultant; and Rod Colvin of Addicus Books, my publisher.

PART I

Nature Meets Nurture:

Partners in

Beauty

Listen to your skin.

Hear it tell you what it needs

at all moments, in all situations.

Give it the personalized attention

and care that it deserves.

—OLIVIER COURTIN-CLARINS, M.D.

chapter 1

Evolution of the Courtin Concept

⌇

O NE OF MY EARLIEST, MOST VIVID MEMORIES is of myself as a child—locking myself in my bedroom and setting off on a marvelous scientific adventure. There, all alone with a wondrous collection of mysterious creams arrayed before me, I would slowly open several of the many jars, carefully scoop out handfuls of their cool, smooth, fragrant potions, and meticulously drop the glorious globs into a large mixing bowl.

Open. Scoop. Drop. Mix.

No two combinations were ever quite the same. A little "mad chemist" was being born. The concoctions fascinated me. I diligently compared their fragrances, textures, odors, and colors with the results of previous secret sessions, making mental notes, quickly designating my favorites and those I liked least. Time and again my parents would bang on the door, demand admittance, and scold me for wasting the valuable products. But I always returned to my experiments. Until well into my adolescent years, I rarely missed an opportunity to sneak back into that captivating world of sweet, soft, beautiful blends.

Far from wasting anything, I was setting the stage for a lifelong passion, a mission of helping women and men look and feel their best. And I would carry on the family tradition. My father was the founder of Clarins, the French cosmetics firm that started as the germ of an idea in an industrious young man's mind and in fifty years has grown into a renowned international group. The creams I so loved as a boy were his creations, which he lovingly called "my babies."

All the while feigning disapproval at my seemingly playful use of those precious concoctions, my parents realized I was onto something, and finally followed my lead. They drafted the whole household into service. Soon everyone was testing my father's products for real. They applied and evaluated them. Most of all, they enjoyed them, although, I am sure, never as much as did I!

Today, thanks to those countless engrossing hours in my bedroom "laboratory," all I need do is touch a skin cream to know if it will do a good job. Far from diminishing over time, my zeal for the contents of those wondrous jars—and their modern-day versions—has never ceased to grow. But my path on the quest for splendid skin took an interesting detour: by way of brittle bones.

World War II put an end to my father's medical studies. After the war, he remained in the sphere of caregiving, launching France's first postsurgical massage-therapy center, where he gradually introduced patients to soothing, healthful creams he made from plant extracts in collaboration with chemical engineers. But he regretted not having returned to school, and pinned his hopes on me: He convinced me to become a doctor.

On Becoming a Physician

Surprisingly, I did not choose to specialize in dermatology. I wanted to make a difference in my patients' health and lives, and, at the time, dermatology offered too few concrete cures. I turned instead to orthopedic surgery, with an emphasis on sports injuries. (While I treated both men and women of all ages, I will focus here on my female patients, as it is for women that I have initially developed my line of customized skin-care products.)

During my years of medical practice, I was struck by the fact that no two patients' needs were identical. Each injury was unique. Each body reacted differently to trauma, treatment, and therapy. Care, therefore, needed to be individualized accordingly. Although some of their injuries were the results of everyday accidents, such as slipping on a staircase or sidewalk, or falling off a step stool, the majority of my patients were either semiprofessional athletes or very avid amateur sportswomen, and had hurt themselves working out or competing. In my practice, many sports and physical activities were represented: aerobics, bicycling, classical and modern dance, fitness training, ice-skating, running, skiing, swimming, tennis, and others.

While treating these women, I could not help noticing that, as much as they went all out for their sport—with no demand being too great as long as it would help them accomplish their athletic or exercise goals—they often either neglected their skin or actually caused it harm. Some had been too busy focusing on workouts and competitions (and, once they had injured themselves, on their resultant pain and subsequent treatment and recovery) to spend time and energy on cleansers, toners, creams, masks, sun protection, and other elements of even the most basic skin-care regimen.

My Early Focus on Skin-Care

Many were involved in outdoor sports, which put them on the front lines for overexposure to sun, extreme cold, pollution, and sometimes even hard, gritty sand. The swimmers were poisoning their skin with chlorine while the skiers were whipping their skin with excessive wind. Others were eating exceedingly unbalanced diets—heavy on pasta, for instance (carbohydrates for the energy to make it to the marathon finish line), but light on or totally lacking in fruits and vegetables. It's these fruits and vegetables that combat free radicals—the atoms responsible for cell damage that results in premature aging.

All of this was complicated by the cycle of skin-related changes through which every woman passes within her lifetime, including those due to the natural aging process.

Yet I was convinced that if my patients' skin looked better, they would feel better—which might hasten their recovery. So once again I plunged into study. Through research, interviews with patients and colleagues, seminars, and extensive reading, it became clear to me that skin changes radically according to a person's age; hormonal state; degree of emotional well-being and stress; nutrition; exercise and sleep habits; level of health or illness and accompanying medications/treatments; and lifestyle in general. I confirmed that skin is affected as well by environmental factors including pollution, type and intensity of sunlight, and weather conditions such as extreme cold and wind.

I also spent a considerable amount of time studying plants, their extracts, and their curative effects on skin. The more I studied, the more I realized that, despite literally millennia of knowledge about and use of plants, they still hold resources and benefits we have yet to discover!

Given my enduring interest in skin and skin care because of my family's business, and now my increasingly deepening knowledge about the science of skin, I began using part of my sessions with patients to focus on their skin. I advised them to "nourish their skin from within" through proper nutrition. I told them about the toxic effects on skin of smoking, substance abuse, insufficient sleep, stress, pollution, and overexposure to sun and winter climate. I continuously reminded them that a positive attitude is the first place to start in treating any part of their body.

My patients knew that their bodies—and minds—needed every available resource and reinforcement to prepare for, undergo, and recover from surgery, and to face what would often be a protracted rehabilitation process. To their great delight, they learned that heeding my suggestions would yield a double payoff. As I always say, "What is good for your skin is usually good for all of your body's parts and systems."

As my attention to my patients' skin grew, however, so did my frustration. I wanted to supplement this "lifestyle advice" with skin-care products, but despite the vast choice of excellent creams for sale, none seemed adaptable to each individual's constantly shifting dermatological needs.

Realizing the Importance of Individualized Skin-Care

The solution, of course, was to custom-make my own product for each patient. Starting with appropriate high-quality creams already on the market, chosen according to each woman's skin type (dry, oily, or combination), I prescribed specific supplements. These consisted of plant extracts, blended in by pharmacists and selected for the properties that would give each woman what her skin uniquely required. Some plant extracts were aimed directly at the skin: to moisturize, tone, or firm, for example; some—by fighting free radicals, reducing inflammation, stimulating and protecting the immune system, providing vitamins and minerals—were intended to help a woman's skin by fortifying her entire system.

In the weeks and sometimes months before their surgery, I asked my patients to apply their personalized creams not only to their faces but also to the areas of their bodies on which I would be operating—

their knees or shoulders, for instance—in order to prepare their skin for optimal healing once it had been cut during surgery. During each appointment I would reassess their skin-care needs and I would modify their custom-made creams accordingly.

But I did not stop there. During their surgical operations, and with their prior consent, I took small samples of their skin, one from the area treated with the custom-made creams, and one from an untreated area. I examined the samples in a laboratory. What I saw was notable: With the use of their individualized creams, my patients' skin-cell structure significantly improved. But I did not have to look through the lens of a microscope to notice the improvement—all I needed to do was see the women themselves.

Their skin looked younger, less dry, more radiant. The wrinkles, creases, lines, and grooves caused by ill-aligned cell layers had begun to smooth out as cells realigned. And their incisions healed quickly and well.

More than ever, I was persuaded that product customization would be of great help for the skin-care needs of women—of all ages, under all environmental conditions, in all life stages and circumstances. This became my dream, my focus, and my goal. But I would have to wait more than a decade for the dream to become reality.

Refining My Skin-Care Beliefs

In 1984, my father asked if I would join in managing the family business. Although I loved practicing medicine, the "little boy in the bedroom laboratory" could not resist the call to work with and among his treasured creams. I started at the company part time, went back to school for an MBA, and in 1995 became executive director of Clarins, the Paris-based cosmetics company. In conjunction with our research and development director Lionel de Benetti, my initial major act was establishing a global network of private and public researchers who would provide the steady stream of active ingredients—including plant extracts—that we required.

The first Clarins product I created was Eclat du Jour—Energizing Morning Cream. Until the launch of the Clarins MEN line in 2002, Eclat du Jour was my favorite product. A throwback to my medical days, it provides all the vitamins the skin needs, and can be of great help to a wide range of women.

Quite ironically, it was this very concept—a treatment formula that performs excellently for nearly everyone—that provided added inspiration toward my dream of another approach to skin care: customization.

As I contemplated what the optimal skin-care treatment might be, my thoughts always returned to the same notions: combining, mixing, harmonizing; combining biotechnology's modern marvels and nature's bounteous riches; mixing the most effective parts of each plant—roots, seeds, stems, leaves, flowers; harmonizing what you inherit from nature with how you enhance it through nurture. A personalized line would need to be built upon the rock-solid basis of what I had learned by living and working with Clarins products: "nourish" a woman's skin by blending vitamins and minerals directly into a cream and be aware that the most efficient products are those that directly meet a clearly defined skin-care need.

The Courtin Concept

The concept that has taken decades for me to refine can now be articulated: For good skin care at any age you must look at your whole body and take care of yourself inside and out, being aware of all influences that could damage your skin and health. As a woman, your skin-care needs are constantly changing, based on many factors. Consequently, your skin-care regimen must be individualized and customized to meet these changes.

Now, isn't it time to listen to your skin and give it personalized attention and care?

chapter 2

To Every Woman There Is a Season: Good Skin Care at Every Age

CAN YOU GUESS HOW LONG your skin cells last? The answer: twenty-five days. What happens after each cell expires? It renews itself, of course. But, as you age, your cells do not regenerate as quickly as they used to, and the new cells are of increasingly diminished quality.

It is important to keep in mind that the skin is not simply the material in which your organs, tissues, and systems are wrapped. The skin is itself an elaborate organ. It's also the body's largest organ. If the skin of an adult were stretched out, it would cover almost two square yards and weigh eight or nine pounds.

Your skin is also part defense system, protecting your network of muscles, bones, nerves, and blood vessels from injury and invasion. It is also part waterproofer—it prevents extreme increases or decreases in body moisture. Your skin is also a sunshade that shields you from dangerous ultraviolet rays. The skin's intricate network of small blood vessels cools you when you overheat, its fat cells insulate you against the cold, and its sweat glands help eliminate waste products and regulate body temperature. The skin even acts as its own doctor, with amazing self-healing capacities rushing to the rescue when you're wounded.

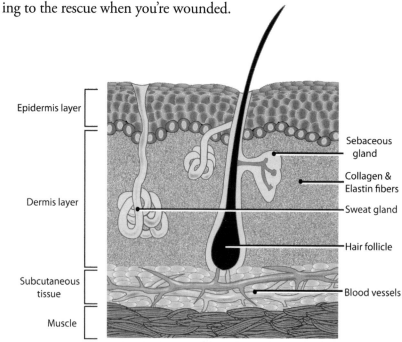

Epidermis layer

Dermis layer

Subcutaneous tissue

Muscle

Sebaceous gland

Collagen & Elastin fibers

Sweat gland

Hair follicle

Blood vessels

The connective tissues, collagen and elastin, are found in the dermis layer of the skin. The health of the collagen determines the contour of the skin and how wrinkled and lined it is. Elastin is responsible for the skin's elasticity.

Your skin is part factory, producing substances such as collagen and elastin, both connective tissues, which help hold skin structures in place. The word "collagen" comes from the Greek and means "glue-producing." A structural protein that makes up 75 percent of your skin, collagen is the body's connective tissue, scaffolding, and blueprint all rolled into one. Like glue, it holds your body together. It also controls cell differentiation and shape. It makes wounds heal and mends broken bones. Elastin, the connective tissue that gives your skin its elasticity, works along with collagen to keep tissues firm and healthy. As the body's supply of collagen and elastin diminish, wrinkles develop.

You don't have to be a scientist, dermatologist, or cosmetician to know that the skin of a twenty-year-old woman does not look or feel like that of her grandmother, her mother, and, often, even her older sister. There's no mistaking the disparities in smoothness, firmness, elasticity, radiance, and uniformity of hue. But do you know *why* these changes happen as you pass through life's different phases? And do you know that, your skin being an extremely complex organ, these are metamorphoses due to psychological and behavioral as well as physical factors? Most importantly, do you know that far from staying on the sidelines as a helpless bystander, observing and lamenting your own aging process, in most cases you can counteract each specific, unique, life-stage-related skin-care challenge?

Three major factors determine your skin's physical appearance: your genes, your lifestyle, and your skin-care regimen. Of course you cannot alter your genetic composition. But it is within your power as to how you take care of yourself in general and your skin in particular. Throughout these pages you will find a detailed presentation of just how you can do this by harnessing the forces of positive attitude, stress management, good nutrition, proper exercise, sun protection, and personalized products—for an all-time, all-out defense against the natural and environmental assaults on your skin.

For now, join me on a quick trip through the three main phases of every woman's life, with a look at how each impacts your skin's needs—whatever your skin type. We'll also examine tips for actively keeping your skin healthy and beautiful all along the way.

Phases of a Woman's Life

Phase 1: Ages Twenty to Thirty

What's Happening Physically?

Young skin possesses a seemingly miraculous ability to quickly repair, renew, and revitalize itself by continually replacing damaged, worn-out tissue. When your skin cells are harmed, an "emergency squad" is set in motion, with neighboring cells dividing more quickly to restore overall cell density and health to normal levels.

However, that does not mean that your skin is being any less assaulted by the ravages of external forces, such as toxic air pollution, the aging effects of overexposure to sun, and the drying effects of severe wind and extreme cold. Your skin is also affected by the "emotional pollution" of stress, or the guaranteed negative results of poor nutrition, insufficient exercise, inadequate sleep, and unhealthful-lifestyle activities such as smoking, drinking, and drug use.

All of these unhealthful forces produce *free radicals*. Perhaps you have heard of free radicals before, but in case you're not totally sure about what they are, let's review with this quick biology lesson. A free radical is an atom with at least one unpaired electron. In the body, this is a molecule that will stabilize itself by stealing an electron from a nearby molecule. When the "attacked" molecule loses its electron, it in turn becomes a free radical, beginning a chain reaction. It is this process that can lead to cell damage and cause aging, cancer, and other diseases.

What Are Your Skin-care Needs?

Because young skin's self-healing capacities are at their peak in this age group, right now you should be concentrating almost exclusively on skin-care products that protect you from further damage, rather than on those designed to do Mother Nature's repair work for her. Women of all ages need to pay strict attention to protecting their skin at all times by using customized products and proper nutrition.

Free radicals are atoms that cause cell damage, which can lead to aging and various diseases. The body's defenses against this process are antioxidants, which interact with the free radicals to prevent cell damage from occurring. Four key antioxidants include: Vitamin C, vitamin E, beta-carotene, and selenium, all of which are found in healthful diets that include fruits, vegetables, and proteins.

What's Happening Psychologically and Behaviorally?

"The young are permanently in a state resembling intoxication," wrote Aristotle. What this and countless similar quotations have in common is the answer to why young skin sometimes looks old: At this time of your life, you think you're invulnerable to the insults that age eventually casts at every woman's skin. And in the psychological sense, you are. The phenomenon to which you're currently *most* invulnerable is the very notion of what it means to get old! It's not that you reject ignore, or deny the idea; you merely have no experience with it—so you cannot imagine yourself as ever being old. "No man knows he is young while he is young," writes Gilbert Keith Chesterton.

If you are young, chances are probably slim that you are even thinking about doing anything for your skin today (using the right products, living a healthful lifestyle) that will stand it in good stead at present and even better stead in future years, when your skin will need more tender loving care. Why worry about wrinkles you'll have in ten years when ten weeks seems so far away?

Of course, no one is asking you to "grow up" too quickly—youth is a time for taking risks, for testing one's limits, for exploring one's world. I agree with Robert Louis Stevenson's words, "Youth is wholly experimental." No, living like your wise old great aunt is not the answer. But it is never too early to gather as much knowledge as possible about the threats your skin faces today and will face tomorrow—and to make optimal use of the right products for confronting those threats.

There's another reason women in this age group often short-change their skin—a reason much less philosophical and much more materialistic: Quality skin-care products are often a financial luxury for young people just staring out in their careers. Unfortunately, in certain cases, you really do get what you pay for—and skin care is among the most glaring examples of that reality. Although there are domains where a bargain product works just as well as its high-end counterpart, skin care is not one of them. The costs of rigorous research and painstaking development that go into creating and producing effective, safe skin-care products are necessarily passed on to the consumer. Though it may take some creative budgeting and a bit of sacrifice in other areas, applying the best products, suited to your personal, specific needs, has to be a priority for women at every stage of their lives.

Phase 2: Ages Thirty to Forty
What's Happening Physically?

In French we say *Plus ça va, moins ça va*. This can be translated as "The further along things go, the less well they go." I always think this expression was coined with our skin in mind!

Just as the robust capacity for self-repair characterizes the skin of twenty- to thirty-year olds, the loss of some of this capacity is one of the most salient changes experienced by women in the thirty-to-forty-year-old group. The ability to self-repair is not totally gone, but it now needs outside help—and it will continue to diminish steadily, and relatively rapidly, with the passage of time. To be more specific, your body now produces lower quantities of the material used for those repairs, substances such as keratin, the fibrous-protein structural units for many living tissues; fibroblasts, the connective-tissue cells that make and secrete collagen proteins; enzymes such as melatonin, which in low concentrations can stimulate skin-cell growth; and anti-oxygenic enzymes, which fight free radicals in your cells.

And don't forget that as you get older there is more to repair. As you age, you have been exposed to more sun, wind, cold, and pollutants, and have experienced more stress and probably eaten more chocolate bars than a woman half your age.

What Are Your Skin-care Needs?

The emergency self-repair squad gets into gear more slowly at this age, with fewer resources at its disposal. Therefore, in addition to using products that protect your skin, you should be focusing on ways to regularly stimulate, encourage, assist, and support the biological substances and mechanisms that renew and revitalize it. This is done through a combination of customized-care products; massage (by yourself or in a treatment salon); excellent, skin-friendly nutrition (which you will read about later in this book); and a strong dose of positive thinking thrown in for good measure!

As far as taking care of yourself in general and your skin in particular, in this age group you have the greatest psychological advantage. You are past the stage when, believing you'll be young forever, you think you do not need to lift a finger to help Mother Nature do her spectacular job. You have not yet entered the stage during which you are increasingly frustrated by the war between Mother Nature and Father Time; this is often a time when you are ready to wave the white flag, surrender, leaving your skin-care products, fresh veggies, and jogging shoes behind. If you are a mother, your children are likely old enough that they do not demand as much of your time. And you are probably far enough along in your professional life that you have the time and the budget for that occasional facial massage; you also probably make sure you don't run out of high-quality skin-care products containing those ingredients you feel will most benefit your skin.

By this point in your life you also know that these privileged years will not last forever. Take advantage of them and do all you can to protect and preserve the health and beauty of your skin.

Phase 3: Age Forty to Fifty and Beyond

What's Happening Physically?

In addition to your skin's having been bombarded by decades of pollution—both environmental and emotional in the form of stress—these are the years of pre-menopause and menopause, and talking about menopause means talking about hormones. Hormones play an essential role in the proper functioning of all cells, especially those in your skin. During this time, your body produces progressively less of the hormones estrogen and progesterone.

A hormone is a substance secreted by a gland or organ and then carried by the bloodstream to tissues on whose metabolism (biochemical processes) it exerts an effect. Just as a television needs an antenna—a receiver—in order to pick up the signal "telling it" to broadcast, a cell has an antenna-like receptor that, from a given molecule, picks up a signal telling the cell to perform a given function—the function of self-repair in skin cells, for example.

Some of these receptors, located inside the cell, are activated by hormones, which must be able to penetrate the cell in order to get the job done. But when hormone production diminishes with age, the fewer existing hormones have more and more trouble working their way into the cell—the opposite of "strength in numbers." Fewer and fewer receptors are thus activated, which means fewer and fewer functions vital to the health and beauty of your skin are performed.

The negative cycle has now been set in motion. As your epidermis, the surface layer of the skin, becomes thinner, your skin becomes more transparent and fragile; it is more vulnerable to attack from the usual suspects—pollution, sun, and extreme weather conditions. Your skin may also become coarser. Gravity as well as diminished collagen and elastin levels cause it to sag. Your blood-vessel walls have also thinned, bringing your blood closer to the surface, causing you to bruise more easily. As we age, the skin weakens further, and so it goes.

> *Your skin loses collagen and elastin and becomes less firm as you age. This occurs first around the eyes and later around the jaw line. The first signs of aging typically appear in your thirties and forties, depending on how well you've taken care of your skin.*

All women need products that protect their skin. In this age group, with your body's factories and supply chains running at progressively slower and less efficient rates, you also need products that replace those missing components. Your skin-care regimen should include ingredients that act like, or play the role of, the hormones that you are no longer producing in sufficient quantity. It should supply molecules that make your cell membranes more permeable, and thus your cells' receptors more accessible for activation. And it should provide from the outside of the collagen, elastin, proteins, peptides, and other components that are no longer abundant enough on the inside.

In most cases your hormone levels do not take precipitous falls. Your collagen supplies do not diminish overnight. These are gradual, progressive, ongoing developments that usually occur over the course of many years. Thanks to the flexibility and convenience of product personalization, you can adapt your skin-care regimen to your body's timing and rhythm, blending in the ingredients you need as your body, in effect, reduces them.

As recently as a generation or two ago, a menopausal woman was considered old. This was partly due to biology, since people lived shorter lives, and partly due to cultural beliefs about what was acceptable behavior for a woman. Once a woman reached the age of fifty, it was assumed she was going downhill psychologically and physically. Fortunately these antiquated notions have become obsolete. Today, many grandmothers wear trendy clothing, run marathons, have active sex lives, divorce, flirt, remarry (sometimes long-lost childhood sweethearts), and own drawers full of "Age is for cheese!" T-shirts.

These are not the grandmothers I worry about.

Another group of middle-aged women are the reigning queens of a self-fulfilling prophecy. They see a little bulge in their belly, say "Well, that's inevitable at my age," and—reasoning that at this point they've lost any possible chance of ever being thin—proceed to eat their way to a bigger bulge in their belly, one that they are then too discouraged ever to get rid of. In the mirror they catch sight of a wrinkle, say "Well, that's inevitable at my age," proceed to do nothing about it, and—when it blossoms into many wrinkles—feel vindicated for not having spent money on face creams in the first place.

However, as the following chapter reminds us, the most important beauty treatment is your brain! With even a modicum of will, discipline, resolve, and ability to get your priorities straight, you can live your life according to that inspiring saying: Age is for cheese!

The human body in all its complexity is often compared to a computer. And just as computers contains files and subfiles and often sub-subfiles, each life stage's biological and psychological consequences reflect the sub-consequences of even minor biological and psychological events that occur within that stage. This does not make things any easier on your skin.

Conditions that Stress the Skin

If You Have Acne

What's Happening Physically?

A condition found most often in the twenty- to thirty-year-old age group, acne has several possible causes. These include the use of oral contraceptives (which have artificially modified the male/female hormone balance), sun exposure, and reaction to medication. Genetics can predispose people to acne; our genetics may give us extremely oily skin and/or skin cells so overabundant that they form a "traffic jam," preventing normal sebaceous (oily) secretions from coming to the surface. This action fosters bacteria growth in the blocked pores.

What Are Your Skin-care Needs?

In order to ensure that you do not further harm your skin, you should use only gentle acne treatments. Harsh preparations give the illusion that you're restoring your skin to its pre-acne state, but what you gain by speeding up the cure, you lose by irritating your skin—sometimes beyond repair.

Moreover, through customization of your skin-care lotions, you can ensure that your acne treatment is compatible with the other products you will still be using as part of your regular skin-care routine of protection, stimulation, repair, and/or replacement, according to your age group.

What's Happening Psychologically and Behaviorally?

You are anxious to get rid of your condition—partly because you are probably in the youngest age range under discussion here, and therefore are at your most impatient, and partly because women of any age want their skin to be clear again. You want to do whatever it takes to get rid of those unsightly marks as soon as possible. By using a milder, albeit slower-acting, treatment, your skin will clear up and you will one day likely forget you ever had acne. Otherwise, by using a fast-acting "cure," you will merely be replacing one type of skin damage with another.

If You Are Pregnant

What's Happening Physically?

In addition to the many and diverse hormonal changes that are preparing and allowing your body to carry, nourish, and give birth to another being, you are, as is always pointed out, eating for two. To your skin, this is of crucial importance. Why? Because your skin is the last to be "fed." Once you ingest the nutrients in food, your bloodstream carries them to all the other parts of you before "serving" your skin. With your baby developing inside you, demand for those precious nutrients only increases. Your skin gets the leftovers—if there are any.

What Are Your Skin-care Needs?

While maintaining the skin-care regimen appropriate for your age group, you need to feed—in the literal sense of the term—your skin from the outside, via creams that contain the nutritional elements you would otherwise be getting from your plate but which your unborn baby is now intercepting. Skin-care products can be customized to include these amino acids, vitamins, minerals, and other components essential for your health in general and your skin's health in particular.

Certain molecules can also be blended into personalized creams to help reduce pregnancy-related skin spots. Like age spots, these occur when a hormonal imbalance triggers overactivity of melanocytes, which are melanin pigment cells in skin, hair, and eyes.

What's Happening Psychologically and Behaviorally?

Pregnancy—and rearing young children—often brings on reactions similar to those mentioned for middle-aged women. The fine line between confronting challenges with creativity and surrendering to them with a sense of inevitability is crossed.

There is no question that your body is changing: In a world frantically obsessed with thinness, you are carrying around a progressively more noticeable belly. The bigger it gets, the harder it is to preserve that graceful gait you were always known for—now, plainly put, you walk funny. You sit awkwardly and stand rarely. Your breasts are enlarged.

You haven't worn your favorite skirts, T-shirts, and high-heeled sandals for months. Your skin, as we've said, may bear unsightly blotches and is generally not looking all that good. You appear and act tired. You are overwhelmed by this transformation. You begin to think that you will be this way for the rest of your life. With each passing day you seem to know less and less where to even begin to make yourself look and feel better. The easiest thing to do in this area of your life is nothing. And that's what you're likely to do.

Or, you've just given birth and find that there are not enough hours in the day. Your new baby seems to demand 100 percent of your time and attention—as do your other children if you have any, and your mate. That's 300 percent and counting! The last thing you could possibly imagine doing is taking three extra minutes to exfoliate your skin.

But it is in just such cases when you most need to take care of yourself. Letting yourself go totally will launch you into a spiraling cycle of increasingly sapped self-esteem, confidence, optimism, *joie de vivre*, energy, and, paradoxically, time. (We take longer to get moving when we're "down" than when we are in top or even normal form.) In the pregnancy instance cited previously, you will worry about not putting your best self forward for your mate—and yet you will feel too discouraged to turn the situation around. In the post-delivery instance, you will be resentful that it's all giving and no receiving—and yet you will feel guilty if you don't supply that 300 percent.

You have to understand that during pregnancy and while rearing your young children a little attention to your own needs goes a very long way. Your feeling healthy and beautiful (and just a little bit pampered!) will give you energy and enthusiasm for getting on with the tasks, responsibilities, and challenges confronting you. Pretty soon, you'll find that you're capable of 400 percent!

If You Are Ill

What's Happening Physically?

If you are ill, your body is summoning and channeling all its resources in defense against the illness. If you are taking antibiotics or other medication, your body is gathering and mobilizing all its resources to ensure the equilibrium of the rest of your organism in the face of these foreign molecules now in your bloodstream. If you have been injured, your body is recruiting and dispatching all its resources to heal the wound. If you are recovering from surgery, even elective plastic surgery, your body is marshaling and deploying all its resources to counteract this shock to your system. If you have been diagnosed with cancer and are undergoing chemotherapy, your body is rallying and directing all its resources to defend against the chemicals' poisonous effects.

As I mentioned in the case of pregnancy, your skin is the last to be nourished even under "normal" circumstances. With nutrients doing double duty as foot soldiers against shock, your skin will surely be starved of the vitamins, minerals, amino acids, and other substances it needs to maintain skin health and beauty.

What Are Your Skin-care Needs ?

Because nourishing your skin is not your system's priority when you are ill, your care regimen has to take on that mission, supplementing your regularly used products with highly customized creams containing the nutrients your skin needs at this especially critical period.

What's Happening Psychologically and Behaviorally?

We've seen examples of points in women's lives—notably during pregnancy and early child rearing, and into and beyond middle age—when the task of tending to their health and beauty needs looks so daunting, so futile, that inaction seems the only "action" to take.

Though wrongheaded, it's very common reasoning. This tendency toward inaction is most pronounced when illness or injury strikes.

However, if there is ever a time when you must unquestionably fight those feelings of futility, get the upper hand, and exercise active, vigorous control over how you look and feel, it is when you are in your most weakened state physically (and thus your most discouraged state psychologically), and on throughout the recovery process—no matter how long it takes! As you will see in the following chapter, you have the power to do this.

Some of you may be saying "This is all very interesting, but it does not reflect reality—or, at least, my reality." And you would be right. Although these descriptions of life phases are accurate, they are not necessarily true for all women. In fact, to say that they were the rigid absolute in all cases would be at odds with the very core of *The Courtin Concept*, which recognizes every woman's individuality, and seeks to enhance her distinct positives and diminish her unique negatives. In some instances, a woman of forty or fifty might experience a problem usually associated with very young adults—acne, for example. Or a woman of childbearing age might have inherited a tendency toward prematurely wrinkle-prone skin. And what about the classic case of identical twins who resembled each other when they were younger but whose lifestyles are now so divergent that one (a smoker) has an ashen tinge while her sister (a health-and-fitness buff) is the picture of radiance?

It is for this reason that a different approach to skin care is needed—one in which a woman's age and skin type are merely two of many determinants in her optimal treatment regimen.

PART II

Six Keys to Beautiful Skin

chapter 3

Key One:
Think Yourself Beautiful

⁓

IN FRANCE WE HAVE A WONDERFUL, frequently used expression: to be *bien dans votre peau.* The literal translation is to be "well in your skin" and it means to be comfortable with yourself, at ease, not uptight (itself a skin-related image). When you are not *bien dans votre peau* you are ill at ease, you feel awkward, there's something amiss. As with commonly used expressions in most languages, when we hear this we focus less on the meanings of the individual words and more on the significance of the phrase as a whole. But it's no coincidence that our ancestors who coined the expression used the concept of "skin" as a yardstick of well-being. As you will see a bit later in this chapter, your skin and your brain are close partners—they communicate with each other, reflect each other's moods, and influence each other's conditions. Someone who is or is not "well in their skin" very likely has skin that, either at that particular moment or in general, is or is not well.

My fondness for another expression might surprise you: "It's what's inside that counts." This might seems strange coming from someone who spends his life making sure people look their best on the outside—through skin-care products and cosmetics. But to its conventional meaning—that true "beauty" comes from the heart—I add the undeniable certainty that if you want to be beautiful, the place to start is not at the cosmetics counter of your local department store, the dress shop, the hair salon, or the gym. The place to start is inside you—more specifically, in your brain. If you do not believe you are beautiful, if you do not believe that you possess the potential to be beautiful, then no product, program, treatment, tool, or bauble-buying spree will make a difference.

Your Mind Is Your Personal Canvas

Nature performs her marvelous artwork through the physical and mental gifts that she gives you at birth and renews all during your life. You optimize those gifts in many ways: by what and how you eat, the kinds of activities in which you engage, the way you manage environmental and emotional onslaughts such as pollution and stress. You nurture them with products, treatments, and other resources from the world around you. But your personal canvas—your brain—must first and foremost be prepared to accept that artwork. Only if you have confidence in yourself, in your innate beauty and in your capacity to continuously become more beautiful, can you be the true, unspoiled reflection of all that nature intended you to be, and of all that nurture helps you become. Only then will the artwork be deeply absorbed into your fibers, and remain there for your pleasure and that of those around you.

Mind–Body Connection

One of the most dynamic and influential proponents of this mind–body reality—indeed, a pioneer who articulated what at the time seemed a revolutionary concept in the Western world—was Dr. Maxwell Maltz. In the middle of the twentieth century, Dr. Maltz had a thriving cosmetic and reconstructive facial-surgery practice. The many patients who came to him were convinced that a new, improved face would be the answer to their problems: that shortening their nose would reduce their anxieties and insecurities, that removing a scar would remove their unhappiness at the same time. Dr. Maltz was initially convinced of this as well. But time and again his patients emerged from their "successful" operations as self-doubting and despondent as before. The now beautiful young woman still felt like the ugly duckling. The accident victim, no longer disfigured, continued to fear leaving his house.

Dr. Maltz thus came to realize that as a result of often invalid perceptions buried in our subconscious from early in life, many of us have inaccurate views of ourselves that limit our potential for personal growth, happiness, success, and beauty—and that no amount of physical cutting and remolding can undo this perception. The remolding, he observed, has to take place in our minds: The "inner scars" have to heal before the "outer scars" can be truly invisible.

From this observation was born Dr. Maltz's breakthrough self-improvement theory and greatly effective "success-conditioning" techniques, presented in his seminal 1960 book *Psycho-Cybernetics*. The nonprofit Psycho-Cybernetics Foundation estimates that 30 million copies of his book have been sold worldwide, and the book has spurred innumerable similar works by psychologists, business leaders, motivation experts, and related professionals.

Dr. Maltz's techniques have been largely used to encourage athletes to make more baskets and touchdowns, and salespeople to close more deals; however, they were inspired by and are of invaluable help to people who cannot fully accept or believe in their own physical beauty until their minds give them "permission" to do so. We've all known the insecure office wallflower who meets the man of her dreams and then suddenly feels—and, most amazingly, even looks!—glowingly beautiful. Or the recent graduate who gets a great job and immediately seems to have grown two inches taller. And what about that friend whose mere decision to start taking better care of herself appears to have produced overnight improvements.

It's not vitamins or makeup artists working overtime here, as involved as they may be in the process. It's the brain that's the paramount vitamin and makeup artist, some have said. This sounds so simple that many women may think it's not worth mentioning. Far from it!

In Asia, such thinking has been a guiding principal for millennia: Tohei Koichi Soushu, a modern-day Japanese aikido master, instructs, "Mind and body were originally one... When we unify our mind and body and become one with the universe, we can use the great power that is naturally ours." Your mind can be your body's greatest ally in your campaign for healthy, beautiful skin.

Have you ever asked a shopkeeper "How's business?" and received the response, "Lousy! Worst year I've ever had! Thinking of closing up forever!" The first thing you'd probably do if you heard that would be to look for an alternative shop. Who wants to give money to—or even be around—a down-in-the-dumps underachiever? And then once you stopped going to that shop, business would be that much worse, which would lead to an even more negative answer from the shop owner when the next person asked the question—which would chase that person right out the door just as quickly. Get the picture?

A more positive reply from the merchant, like "Great!" or even a mild "OK!" thrusts the self-fulfilling prophecy into positive territory. You feel confident in the shop, you keep coming back, passersby see customers in the store so they feel encouraged to enter as well. Several years ago, although not suffering a downturn, the well-known French hypermarket company Carrefour went one step further and created a motto—splashed all over its advertising in huge red and white letters—that translates to "With Carrefour, I positivize!" It doesn't get more stirring than that!

Beauty Is the Supreme Self-Fulfilling Prophecy

Try this easy experiment: As you close your eyes at night—when you're in that hazy zone between totally awake and totally asleep—envision yourself as the healthiest, happiest, most beautiful you could want to be. In this vision, place yourself in a setting that represents the height of relaxation, gratification, pleasure, or excitement: on a tropical beach, for instance, or at a holiday dinner surrounded by all those you hold dear. Or maybe looking out over glamorous Paris from the top of the Eiffel Tower. Silently repeat, "I am healthiest. I am happiest. I am most beautiful. I am healthiest. I am happiest. I am most beautiful." Let the full meaning of these words profoundly penetrate your consciousness. In the scene in your mind, see the "you" as the ultimate you—all you have ever hoped for, and more! Focus on this image and repeat the words and repeat them and repeat them, until you have fallen asleep. Then focus and repeat them the following night, and the nights after. And right before you get out of bed every morning, focus and repeat them again.

After just a week has passed, see how *bien dans votre peau*—"well in your skin"—you feel, in the figurative and literal meanings of the term. Better still, see how even more motivated and ready you are to set off on an active program of making sure you feel—and thus look—your best for the rest of your life! Then don't be surprised if others start saying, "I can't put my finger on it, but there's something different about you." "Are you in love? You look great!" "What's your secret?"

In its general role as "gatekeeper" to your attitude about your own beauty, the brain has a particularly interesting relationship with your skin. I said at the beginning of this chapter that the brain and the skin are close partners, communicating with each other, reflecting each other's moods, influencing each other's conditions. Working as part of a cohesive team, where each member plays an equally important role, they communicate with you as well, sending you messages that are easy to pick up, interpret, and use to your advantage—if you know what to look for.

Among the team's loyal messengers are your nerve endings—which carry out obvious functions like directing your brain to tell you to pull your hand away when you touch a hot stove, or to jump back onto dry land when the tips of your toes venture into the icy ocean. But they also perform such magic as instructing your brain to make your skin feel tight, or tingly, or itchy, when you're in situations of extreme emotion, like waiting to be interviewed for the job you've always wanted, finding yourself in the cafeteria line next to the person you have a crush on, or knowing that you're about to be caught in a lie.

In collaboration with your senses of smell and sight, your nerve endings can play tricks on you, too—for example, leading you to think a neutral lotion is a sunblock just because it feels, smells, and looks like the most popular sunblock in the stores. Or, as in some scientific experiments, making you believe a heat-generating, medicinal-smelling gel purported to soothe your irritated skin has in fact done so although the item is a placebo.

At work here is "sense memory." This is what makes a golden oldie on the radio suddenly catapult you back to how you felt the first time you heard it and why the smell of cotton candy immediately evokes visions of a carnival. Sense memory's undeniable power has been successfully harnessed by the burgeoning aromatherapy industry, whose fragrant inhalants, creams, and lotions seek to influence your mood, producing the sensation (and thus often the reality) of peace, well-being, and good health.

Focus on the pleasure skin-care products bring, thanks to your brain and its distinct set of messengers. After all, pleasure is what beauty is about. You might be so busy observing the primary effects of personal-care products—the way they look on you or make you look—that you don't realize how many secondary delights they offer: the smooth cool kiss of a cream as it slides along your forehead; a lotion's pleasant scent, which seems so appropriate to its purpose; even the beautiful colors and shapes of the packaging. But perhaps the most important service your brain-skin connection can provide is its highly sophisticated alarm system. Afflictions such as acne, psoriasis, eczema, inflammation, shingles, and the vast category of conditions generally referred to as "rashes" are red flags alerting you that something is wrong. Possibly it's something in your immune system, or perhaps it's due to emotional/stress overload, or maybe it's in the way your body is reacting to the free radicals in our environment. Or it could be any number of other factors.

In your goal of being *bien dans votre peau,* listen to your skin first and foremost by listening to your inner-most thoughts.

chapter 4

Key Two:

Beware of Your Skin's Enemies:
Pollution and Stress

HAVE YOU EVER LIVED IN A HOUSE with "white" walls and then, after many years, had them repainted white? Most likely, to your absolute astonishment, when the first drop of the fresh coat of paint was applied, the old "white" paint suddenly seemed so yellow—almost beige—in comparison. You asked yourself how you could have been so wrong about the color.

The answer of course is that you were not wrong at all. Dust, general household dirt, pollution, possibly cigarette smoke—to say nothing of little children brushing against the walls on their way out to play—yellowed the paint so gradually, by such minuscule increments, that you never noticed the change.

So it is with two negative influences that affect you day in and day out, hour in and hour out: pollution and stress. Although one attacks from the outside in and the other from the inside out, I group them here because, without realizing it, you become so used to their battering, to the gradual, subtle, constantly increasing intensity with which they unremittingly chip away at your health and well-being, that you no longer even notice them as they change your "white" walls.

Although it's a much-simplified image of extremely complex phenomena, the "partnership" of pollution and stress can be pictured like this: Pollution is produced in the environment outside you—in the air you breathe—and hits you first and foremost on the inside, doing damage to the cells that constitute your skin. While that damage very soon appears where you can see it—in wrinkles, dryness, ashen or yellowy color, blemishes, premature aging—for a while you remain unaware of the poisonous processes going on.

Stress is generated in the environment inside you—in your central nervous system—and hits you unmistakably on the outside, aggravating or activating conditions such as acne, blisters, cold sores, eczema, hives, itchiness, psoriasis, rosacea, warts, and signs of aging. While the damage is necessarily occurring within your cells, the effects are almost immediately visible when you look in your mirror. And let's face it: As much as we care about the medical and scientific aspects of our skin—facts and figures concerning cell structure, blood-vessel activity, and the frightening effects of free radicals, for instance—what most inspires us to start and maintain a skin-care regimen is the way our skin looks.

Operating together, as they do in most modern lives, pollution and stress form a tenacious force laying siege to your skin from all directions. It is easy, especially given our increasingly rushed lives, to do only the minimum—if even that—to defend and reinforce our skin against perils such as pollution and stress. But in the long run that is definitely not the best course. The best—and easiest—path is to do all you possibly can to nurture your skin. As I said in the previous chapter, good skin-care rituals are brimming with many obvious benefits—not the least of which are improvements in the way you look and thus feel, and the general satisfaction of knowing that you are taking great care of yourself. And they are full of many delightful bonuses as well—such as the silken textures and pleasant fragrances of the products you use, and even the artistry of their packaging. What could be more pleasant and easier to handle than that?

Although it seems counterintuitive, the more difficult move is to do nothing, or to do only the bare minimum. Even if you do a lot, if the products you use are not suited to your specific, unique needs, they will be ineffective at best, and risk irreparable damage to your skin at worst. If abuse is piled upon abuse, one day in the not too distant future you will wake up with as many regrets as wrinkles, and with your skin tone as dreadful as your morale. To mount the best defense against the effects of pollution and stress, you have to know how your enemies operate and what the battlefield looks like.

Pollution

Despite all its marvels, the skin is, alas, on the front lines of battle—the first target vulnerable to pollution. The skin absorbs pollutants through its pores and thus allows them to affect other areas of your body.

A pollutant doesn't have to have a fancy name or be an unfamiliar entity to do damage. Even ordinary household and environmental "dust"—in both urban and rural areas—is considered noxious when it raises the number of bacteria on your skin, clogs your pores, and thus gives you unsightly, unhealthful, and often persistent blemishes.

And what is more familiar to human beings than the sun?

Some of you may still remember the days, many decades ago, before it was trumpeted in almost every popular magazine and at almost every cosmetics counter that sun exposure leads to skin damage. Back then, nothing seemed more natural than to spend an entire summer soaking up rays, covered with nothing but the slightest coat of "suntan lotion" purchased at the local drugstore. When wrinkles, blotches, and roughness showed up in short order, women wrote these off as part of the "natural" aging process, about which, they thought, nothing could be done.

We now know that sun exposure is one of the primary causes of premature skin aging—and certainly of skin cancer! The sun's ultraviolet light not only penetrates the outer layer of your skin, but also deeply invades the layers underneath, where the work of keeping your skin toned, supple, and generally healthy takes place. The results are dramatic: The creation of free radicals, wrinkles, blotches, discoloration, roughness, loss of resilience, increased tendency for bruising, lowered immunity against disease and infection, and collagen breakdown—all leading to sagging, uneven texture, and more wrinkles.

Although potential new pollutants are being studied daily by scientists—and a list of the existing menaces looks like a combination of alphabet soup and secret code—the cause-and-effect dirty work of two major categories of culprits has become more familiar to us in recent years through increased attention in the mainstream media: toxic air pollutants and stratospheric-ozone depleters.

Toxic Air Pollutants

Toxic air pollutants hamper your skin's built-in systems for defense, renewal, and repair, leaving it all the more exposed to further, and lasting impairment. They ravage the natural oils that capture and lock in your skin's elasticity-maintaining moisture. Along with other pollutants, such as alcohol, stress, too much exposure to the sun, air pollution causes the occurrence of free radicals—responsible for the breakdown of your skin's cellular structure and for premature aging.

The list of toxic air pollutants is long. Some examples are arsenic, asbestos, benzene, dioxin, methylene chloride, perchloroethylene, toluene, and metals such as cadmium, chromium, lead compounds, and mercury.

Each toxic air pollutant comes from a somewhat different source. Benzene is especially well known as naturally occurring in cigarette smoke, crude oil, and gasoline. It's also recognized for its extensive use in the manufacturing of a wide variety of products, including some types of drugs, pesticides, lubricants, detergents, rubber, dyes, and other chemicals that, in turn, go into synthetic fibers, resins, plastics, and nylon. Many toxic air pollutants are produced in chemical plants or result from the burning of fossil fuels. Perchloroethylene is released from some dry-cleaning facilities.

Certain industries use methylene chloride as a solvent and paint stripper. As with formaldehyde and asbestos, when a pollutant is a component of building materials, indoor air problems may arise.

Environmental and medical professionals endlessly worry about the degree to which toxic air pollutants enter and affect our food and water supply, while botanists, zoologists, and ecologists express concern for their consequences on plants, animals, and indeed our planet itself.

Among their vast range of deleterious consequences (birth defects and eye and respiratory problems, to name a few), toxic air pollutants' effects on the health and beauty of your skin can range from mild irritation to cancer.

Stratospheric-Ozone Depleters

This group comprises such gases as chlorofluorocarbons (CFCs) and other compounds that include chlorine or bromine. Also known as "greenhouse gases," chlorofluorocarbons are chemical substances that drift to the upper stratosphere and erode the earth's protective ozone layer. CFCs are present in fire extinguishers and aerosol cans. Because they perform well as coolants, they are incorporated into air conditioners and refrigerators. Other stratospheric-ozone depleters are used as industrial solvents.

As their category name implies, these chemicals are capable of destroying the ozone in the stratosphere. Ozone plays a major role in absorption of the sun's harmful ultraviolet-radiation (UVB) light. When the ozone layer is depleted, this dangerous ultraviolet radiation penetrates the earth's surface, thereby making us vulnerable to the development of skin cancer, eye problems, and other conditions, and causing harm to animals and plants.

Stress

Some years ago in France there was an amusing commercial in which hundreds and hundreds of sugar cubes had been lined up, standing on their ends, on a large surface with slight peaks and valleys. The row of cubes went on and on. Someone lightly flicked the first cube. It tipped backward into the next, which fell into the next and so on, converting the entire, seemingly endless line into one huge, domino-effect, rolling ripple.

I think of this commercial every time I hear or read the word "stress." The difference being, of course, that stress is not amusing at all.

The domino effect of stress is twofold: first in how it strikes, then in what it does to you—including your skin—once it has hit. When you focus specifically on the evils of stress-generated free radicals—chain reactions in and of themselves—you understand why this scourge demands your urgent vigilance and attention.

Cumulative Effect of Stress

A single stressful incident rarely occurs in isolation. For example, you have a fight with your partner right before leaving for work. There's no time to resolve the conflict so you just turn and dash out the door—in a state of stress. You're so frazzled by the fight that, you suddenly realize, you have forgotten that you're almost out of gas. Now late for work, you stop at a station, where you try to beat another car to the pump. Not only does that car get there first, but you nick its fender in the process. The owner takes your license number and says you'll hear from his insurance company. You zoom away—even later for work and more stressed. Finally when you arrive at the office, your boss makes a snide comment about your need to get a new alarm clock and you spend the rest of the day stressed and obsessing over whether you're about to lose your job. By the time you walk into your home at the end of the day, you are certainly not calmer than you were when you left that morning.

Unfortunately, the chain reaction of stress does not stop with your feelings. While your mind and emotions are churning, your body is being attacked—and in more places than you think. One of the most alarming targets is your immune system, the loyal army that guards and protects you against invasion, infection, and disease. Once stress weakens the immune system's barricades, your entire being is left vulnerable—like a house with its front door knocked down—with each subsequent attack harming an already fragile organism.

If you're looking for someone to blame for the ills stress inflicts on your skin, you can turn to our prehistoric ancestors. It is said that even with all the mind-boggling technological advances humans have made during our approximately three million years of existence, our central nervous systems have not changed significantly in all that time. The "fight-or-flight" mechanism with which our primitive forebears reacted to perceived danger is the same innate, instinctive, automatic response we have to stress today.

Though not a wooly mammoth or a saber-toothed tiger, stress tells our systems that we had better prepare to fight—to summon up the best answers we possibly can on that grueling final exam, for instance.

Stress prompts us to run for safety, figuratively speaking, when we have anxiety about a big meeting or other challenging situation.

During the fight-or-flight response, oxygen, blood, and nutrients are "borrowed" from the parts of your body, such as your skin, not deemed essential for confronting the stress, and rushed to the areas directly involved in the crucial response, such as your adrenal glands and muscles. With chronic stress, your skin is repeatedly deprived—eventually starved—of these vital resources. The results? Your skin has trouble breathing. It is less hydrated and thus less supple and more prone to wrinkling. It looks lifeless and dull. Your pores clog more easily and blemishes form. You look old before your time.

Your skin doesn't escape the effect of stress on digestion, either. Have you ever tried to eat a three-course meal (or even a few crackers) when your stomach was in knots? Even if you could eat, in a stressed state your body does not absorb all the nutrients it is taking in, while at the same time, undigested impurities build up faster than they can be eliminated. Once again, the results can be read on your skin like a book—with a very unhappy ending.

But the most obvious way stress leaves its mark on your face requires the least amount of scientific knowledge or terminology to express. It can be defined in one ordinary word: "grimace." You may prefer "frown," "scowl," or even their milder cousin, "pout." These, and more (sometimes **worse!**), are all the things you do with your face when mental or emotional pressure overtakes you. The step from constantly scrunched-up cheeks, eyes, and forehead to permanently set-in lines and wrinkles is a short one.

What Is a Body (and Face) to Do?

Within the past several decades, advice for combating stress has exploded into a booming industry. There are now countless books, Web sites, seminars, motivational speakers, and magazine articles—not to mention family members, friends, colleagues, and even casual acquaintances—telling you how to de-stress. We hear such things as: get organized, take yoga classes, think positively, make time for yourself once a day, count your blessings upon awakening, take a deep breath before entering your office, turn your car into a buffer zone, luxuriate in the bathtub, or take yourself to the movies.

There is no denying the immeasurable value of such tips and the many others among which to choose. But in responding to the effects of stress on your skin—just as to those of pollution and of meteorological menaces like excessive sunlight, strong wind, and extreme temperatures—words are not enough. These forces cause unhealthy, undernourished, oxygen-starved, dry, wrinkled, blemished, discolored, and old-looking skin. To combat the threat of these problems, you need an excellent and customized skin-care regimen that does the following:

- Brims with super-healthful antioxidants to battle cell damage caused by free radicals.

- Has natural, built-in shields to protect you from the elements.

- Deeply and thoroughly cleanses your skin of impurities; sloughs off dead cells; and prepares your face, neck, and body to receive nourishing, hydrating, revitalizing creams and lotions.

- Has silky textures and fragrant essential oils to comfort you, give you pleasure, make you smile—in other words, reduce your stress.

Above all else, a good skin-care regimen is totally and continually customized for you; it should be based on your age, your skin type, the meteorological and environmental conditions where you live and travel, how you feel, how you eat, and how you live.

chapter 5

Key Three:

Eat, Drink, and Be Beautiful

I T IS SAID THAT IF YOU PUT A BABY ALONE in a room where every possible food is scattered around on the floor—nutritious food and food with "empty calories"—the child will, as if "programmed" by Mother Nature, crawl over to only the wholesome items, one by one, eventually choosing a completely healthful, balanced meal.

Whether this is a universal truth or not, we'd all like to have faith in our natural capacity to take excellent care of ourselves—and taking excellent care of ourselves starts with good nutrition. Of course, in that room with the baby there are no lavishly produced television commercials for the latest luscious sweet-treat, no all-you-can-eat buffets, no mother-in-law complaining that you haven't touched her lasagna, and no little voice whispering, "You worked two weekends in a row to get that report done—you deserve some onion rings!"

We have said that your brain is your greatest ally in your quest for optimum health and beauty. As is the case with following a good skin-care regimen, merely thinking of the rewards of good nutrition (or the penalties of bad nutrition) should be enough to kick your motivation into high gear and keep it there—for the sake of your skin in particular and your body in general. You can be pretty sure that if what you are eating promotes healthy, beautiful skin, it will be good for you overall. And vice versa. As will be seen in later examples, this is especially true when you take in plenty of antioxidants, nature's trusty soldiers in the fight against the aging effects of free radicals.

The opposite of this is true as well: If your body lacks certain nutrients, your skin does not escape the results. Deficiencies of essential fatty acids, A- and B-complex vitamins, and other substances, for example, not only impede your skin's wondrous capacity to repair and revitalize itself, but also can lead to specific skin conditions, such as certain forms of dermatitis.

Drinking water plays a major role in staying healthy. Water helps keep muscles and skin toned, assists in weight loss, transports oxygen and nutrients to cells, eliminates toxins and wastes from the body, and regulates body temperature.

Water: A Key Ingredient

As for the basic healthful eating guidelines, how about this for simplicity: The star headliner on our list for a skin-healthy diet is colorless, odorless, and basically tasteless. It requires no chewing, cooking, or preparation. It has no calories, in its natural state contains none of the fancy-sounding nutrients whose praises I sing in this chapter, and at times it even goes unnoticed on your meal table. This is a shame, because the more you notice it, consume it throughout the day, and go back for seconds, thirds, fourths, and more, the healthier you will be and your skin will look. I am talking, of course, about water. And no discussion of good nutrition should start without it.

Although water makes up about 70 percent of our bodies, the older we get, the less we feel thirsty—and thus, unless we pay focused attention to doing so, the less we drink. It's ironic that water is one of the most vital nutrients in out diets, yet is one of the most neglected. I have heard water referred to as "the forgotten nutrient." Here are just several of many reasons for going out of your way to enjoy one of nature's greatest health and beauty products:

Water naturally rejuvenates your skin. Drinking water prevents dehydration throughout your body. Drinking lots of water—at least eight eight-ounce glasses per day, plus one eight-ounce glass per each hour of light activity—keeps your skin well hydrated, a good step toward helping it stay supple and smooth. Well-hydrated skin may also sag less after weight loss.

Here's an important point to be made about getting enough water daily: Coffee, tea, hot chocolate, and cola contain caffeine, which acts as a diuretic, causing you to eliminate water via urination. If you drink these, do so in addition to your eight glasses of water per day. If you drink them in significant quantities, drink even more water to counteract their diuretic effects. Although drinking plenty of water is important, if you wish to prevent morning puffiness, taper off your intake of water and other fluids two to three hours before bedtime.

As an automobile needs gasoline, and a machine needs oil for its parts, your body needs water in order to perform its countless functions, including digestion, circulation, maintaining muscle tone, and regulating body temperature.

Water flushes waste products from your system. In case you've ever wondered where "cottage cheese" thighs come from, the answer is: waste products in your system.

Water helps burn fat, naturally suppresses appetite, and—paradoxically—gets rid of the excess water that makes you feel heavy. Interestingly, the less water you drink, the more water you retain!

Nutrition Guidelines

The guidelines for nutrition may seem complex, but are actually simple, centering on two key concepts: balance and variety. Eating a balanced, varied diet—including a wide assortment within each recommended food group—ensures that you get the right amounts of all the essential nutrients your body needs. For your body and skin to function properly, they need carbohydrates, proteins, fats, vitamins, and minerals. Balanced nutrition also means getting enough fiber, especially through whole grains and loads of fruits and vegetables.

While a good, balanced diet keeps you healthy, it also is one of the easiest ways to avoid weight gain, which is a bane not only for your overall health and your self-image but also for your skin. Why? Because extra fat stretches the skin and then leaves wrinkles and sagging behind once the extra pounds are lost. It also impedes the flow of oxygen to your skin, leaving it looking pale and lifeless. Finally, fat contains toxins and excessive numbers of adipocytes (fat cells), forming a noxious layer on which your skin must rest.

Daily Food Guide for Adults
U.S. Department of Agriculture

Grains

- Consume 6 to 11 servings of grain foods, breads, cereals, rice, pasta. Whenever possible, choose whole-grain products, for the fiber your system needs for staying in good shape—and thus your skin needs for staying clear and radiant.

Fruits and Vegetables

- Eat 3 to 5 servings of vegetables. (A serving is one-half cup.) The fresher the vegetables, the better. Veritable cornucopias of vitamins, minerals, and antioxidants, vegetables are powerful weapons for fighting the aging effects of free radicals. Favor deep-colored vegetables such as spinach, broccoli, beets, red peppers (many of the pigments that give them color are antioxidants) and cook them as little as possible or not at all; heat inactivates certain antioxidants, removes many vital nutrients from food, and increases its free-radical content.

- Eat 2 to 4 servings of fruit. We derive the same benefits from fruits that we do from vegetables. The deep-colored ones bursting with antioxidant benefits include berries, cherries, oranges, and dried fruit such as raisins and prunes. Juice is fine but only 100 percent fruit juice counts as fruit, and whole fruits are higher in fiber than juice.

Meat and Poultry

- Eat 2 to 3 servings of meat and meat alternatives such as fish, poultry, eggs, dry beans, and nuts. To reduce fat intake, select lean meat and fish, remove skin from poultry, and eat nuts in moderation. Trim away all visible fat before roasting, boiling, or broiling meat. Avoid frying.

Dairy Products

- Consume 2 to 3 servings of dairy products such as milk, yogurt, and cheese. Choose low-fat varieties whenever possible.

Fats, Oils, and Sugars

🐦 Use fats, oils, and sugars sparingly. When cooking and preparing meals, hold back on oil, butter, margarine, cream, mayonnaise, sauces, gravies, dressings (lemon juice is a great dressing stand-in). When shopping, go out of your way to avoid reaching for sugary drinks and for foods high in fat, salt, and sugar. When snacking, think "Substitute! Substitute! Substitute!" Try dried fruit instead of candy, frozen yogurt instead of ice cream, a cinnamon-raisin bagel instead of cookies, sparkling water mixed with 100 percent fruit juice instead of soda.

Remember, although you should use fats sparingly, it is a mistake to avoid them altogether. Our bodies need them for growth, energy, insulation, support and cushioning of organs, regulation of some body processes, transport and absorption of certain vitamins and other nutrients, and maintenance of healthy skin. However, not all fats are alike. There are good fats and bad fats.

Good Fats

🐦 *Polyunsaturated fats* are found in fish and plant sources. Particularly desirable polyunsaturated fats are those found in the cold-water fish like salmon and sardines, which contain omega-3 fats, essential fatty acids. Plant sources of omega-3 fats include flaxseed, soybeans, walnuts, oat germ, raw spinach, wheat germ, and raw broccoli. Flaxseed is a rich source of alpha-liolenic acids, one of the omega-3 fats.

- *Monounsaturated fats* are found in oils such as olive, canola, and sunflower as well as in avocados. These fats do not increase cholesterol levels in the blood.

Bad Fats

- *Saturated fats* are mainly found in animal fats, whole-milk products, and some plant foods, including coconut and coconut oil, palm oil, and palm kernel oil.

- *Trans fats* act like saturated fats. They are produced by heating vegetable oil to a solid state to extend the shelf life of food products, a process known as hydrogenation. The more solid the fat, the more trans fats produced. These hydrogenated fats are found in commercially prepared baked goods, margarine, snack foods, and processed foods. Commercially fried foods, such as French fries, are high in trans fats.

- *Omega-6 fats* come from such foods as vegetable oils and the meat of grain-fed animals. Too much of these fats can increase blood clotting and constrict blood vessels, thereby increasing the risk of heart disease, stroke, and possibly cancer.

Losing Weight

Stay away from fad diets! Any kind of fad eating plan is unhealthful at best, dangerous at worst; what I call the "low-highs" (low-carbohydrate, high-carbohydrate, low-protein, high-protein, and the list goes on and on) are downright frightening from a health-and-beauty standpoint. Continually increasing in type and popularity, these regimes are imbalanced not merely because they favor only one food group and ignore others, but also because they focus on only one kind of result and ignore others. If you do not eat a balanced, varied diet, sure your waistline might decrease under certain conditions, but so will your health—and with it, the radiance, suppleness, and youthful look of your skin.

Why seek to fool your body into weight loss through some "magic formula" of disproportion when, for literally thousands of years, we have been programmed to follow nature's formula for correct eating, which includes, when need be, effective dieting.

This means cutting calories by reducing portion size within a food group and by eliminating "empty-calorie" munchies. But do not cut nutrients by bypassing a food group itself.

TIP FROM DR. COURTIN

Drinking water will help you lose weight. Water contains no calories, and serves as an appetite suppressant.

Eliminate or significantly reduce what your body doesn't need: sugars and trans fats, found in processed foods and especially in snacks. But do not eliminate what your body needs: "good" sugars, found in foods like pasta, rice, whole-grain breads; healthful fats, found in olive oil, nuts, and seafood with its heart-friendly omega-3 fatty acids.

Learn about good nutrition. Read as much as you can about it. Talk to your doctor. Find out which combinations and quantities of foods/ nutrients will help your weight-loss efforts and which combinations and quantities will hinder them. Avoid sugar, smoking, and alcohol. Each causes the production of free radicals. Each carries numerous and various threats to your health as a whole. All have one specific thing in common: They make your skin look old.

Effects of Sugar

To understand the damage sugar does to your skin, you need to understand how simple sugar effects collagen, the important connective tissue that provides the structural foundation of your skin.

Processed sugar and products containing it enter your bloodstream very quickly. When this happens, "glycation" occurs, a reaction that hardens collagen the way the sun hardens a rubber hose left outside too long, or the way the tanning process toughens a hide. Your skin loses its elasticity and its even color. The lines and wrinkles that form when you smile or squint or frown no longer smooth out once you relax your face. Eventually they become deep grooves.

Stop Smoking

Have you ever heard of "smoker's face"? Exclusive to smokers, it's easy to spot. Smokers often have a gaunt look, a grayish tint to their skin along with wrinkles and sagging skin. Even if they smoked only in their teens and twenties, by age forty to fifty smokers have wrinkles comparable to those of nonsmokers twenty years their senior. The longer you smoke, the less remediable this is, especially as smoking impairs the body's natural ability to heal itself and to recover from disease, injury, and surgery. Smokers experience more scarring, as well. Why is this so? The nicotine in cigarettes causes blood vessels to constrict, keeping blood from flowing to the capillaries that nourish the skin.

Seeing only some of the reasons behind "smoker's face" makes us realize that those good-looking models in cigarette ads of yore were certainly not representative of true smokers.

Avoid Alcoholic Beverages

Whatever pleasure alcohol seems to afford our taste buds and state of mind is quickly overshadowed by what it takes away from the rest of our bodies, and our skin is included in the wreckage. Although it's a liquid, alcohol actually dehydrates us. Think of what happens to a leaf when it dries out—it becomes brittle, cracked, wrinkled. Your dehydrated skin suffers the same fate, as well as turning red and blotchy. In addition, by widening the small blood vessels in your skin, alcohol causes increased blood flow to the surface, resulting in that flushed, "broken-vein" look.

Alcohol depletes the body of vitamin B complex and other nutrients crucial for healthy skin. It often interferes with or disrupts healthful eating patterns, leading to malnourishment and all its accompanying woes.

Dangers of Substance Abuse

Substances considered "drugs" may include over-the-counter and prescription medication (whether taken for medical purposes or not) as well as illegal drugs such as marijuana, hashish, cocaine, heroine, hallucinogens, and inhalants. The recent surge in some athletes' use of unsafe, banned, performance-enhancing chemicals, such as steroids, has added another category to this list. The outright abuse of any of these is, at best, perilous for your health in general and for your skin in particular. At worse, it can be lethal.

To add to the dangers, individuals who overindulge in such substances often make the same nutritional mistakes as do smokers and heavy drinkers: They eat inadequately and infrequently. Even excessive coffee intake can produce these results. Varying according to the drug and the amounts taken, potential harm to your skin can include: discoloration, break-outs, and dehydration of not only the skin but also the eyes and other areas of your body. Other side effects may include: infections, abscesses, ulceration, blood spots, bruises, itching, and an accelerated appearance of aging. Not a pretty picture, is it?

Vitamins and Supplements

People's opinions of vitamins and supplements run the gamut. At one extreme are individuals who believe that if you eat healthfully, exercise, get enough sleep, and protect yourself from environmental hazards, you don't need any supplements whatsoever.

At the other extreme are people who load up on so many supplements per day that they practically need a Ph.D. in nutrition, a private warehouse, and special data-base software to keep track of them all—not to mention extra hours in the day to take them all and a small fortune to afford them!

In the middle of the spectrum are those who eat well, take good care of themselves, and take a daily multi-vitamin/multi-mineral capsule. These people are aware of which vitamins, minerals, and other substances benefit their skin. Barring medical conditions that necessitate specially prescribed supplements and nutritional monitoring, this is the best category to be in. It's best to always check with your doctor about which vitamins or supplements are appropriate for you. However, the following basics will give you an overview of vitamins and how they benefit your skin.

Vitamin A: Used in treating acne; seems to smooth out wrinkles and improve texture by restoring the skin's collagen-forming capability.

Vitamin B complex: A full range of B vitamins, including biotin, choline, folic acid, inositol, PABA (para-aminobenzoic acid), and the six "numbered" B vitamins—B-1 (thiamin), B-2 (riboflavin), B-3 (niacin), B-5 (pantothenic acid), B-6 (pyridoxine), and B-12 (cobalamin). B vitamins are important in the maintenance of healthy skin.

Vitamin C: Has antioxidant powers that protect against free radicals, especially those due to sun exposure; contributes to collagen production, thus helps keep skin firm. Excess vitamin C is passed through the kidneys and flushed from the body. Megadoses are dangerous, as they "train" the body to flush out excess after excess, so that soon the flushing mechanism kicks in even when smaller—needed—doses are ingested.

Vitamin E: Claimed to be effective for skin-tissue health—and thus healthy-looking skin; protects against free radicals, especially those due to sun exposure.

Alpha-lipoic acid: A powerful, natural antioxidant—another weapon in the fight against free radicals.

Supplements containing carotenoids: Can help protect against sun-related free radicals.

Fatty acids (such as in fish oil): Help the skin retain moisture—for softness, smoothness, resilience.

Zinc: Can help protect against sun-related free radicals.

It bears repeating: You need both skin care from the outside through the finest customized beauty products, and skin care from the inside through excellent dietary habits. These are two essential members of the high-performance team working for the optimal health of your skin and for the radiant, satisfied smile you will see when you look in the mirror.

chapter 6

Key Four:

Be Sun-Smart

⁓

W HEN IT COMES TO PROTECTING YOUR SKIN from the sun, knowledge is power. What you don't know may lead not only to wrinkles, but also to cancer. Because skin damage from even one occurrence of overexposure can never be reversed, learning about your skin and protecting it must become a lifelong habit. Overexposure to sunlight is one of the most damaging forces to our skin. Further, sun damage is cumulative—it starts in childhood and continues through adulthood. The sun emits two types of damaging ultraviolet rays: UV-B rays, which cause obvious burning of the skin, and UV-A rays that penetrate the skin, weakening collagen and contributing to wrinkling and other signs of age.

In previous chapters I discussed the sun's ultraviolet radiation as an environmental "pollutant," and I highlighted nutrients that help protect your skin from its ravages. I spoke of the necessity to use skin-care products customized for your particular circumstances and your unique needs—including the type and intensity of sunlight to which you are exposed where you live and where you travel. I am sure that much of this sounded familiar to you, since, as we've said, almost every sector of the media today is overflowing with facts, figures, and warnings concerning exposure to the sun. However, these facts, figures, and warnings are sometimes interwoven with myths, some of which have been believed for decades. Fact must be separated from fiction if women are to understand their skin and take control of their individualized skin-care program.

MYTH: A suntan is a symbol of good health.

How interesting that a century ago, having the palest of skin was the height of fashion and an indication of financial comfort. Women with suntans were those who needed to work outside in the fields for a living. Today, having a deep tan is the height of fashion and an indication of financial comfort; women with suntans are those who have the leisure time and disposable income for participating in outdoor sports or going to the beach, on a cruise, or to a tanning salon.

So ask yourself this: Do you drive, or ride as a passenger, with the sun streaming in through the window onto your face, arm, upper body, even—depending on the angle—your legs? Do you walk to and from your house to your car or the bus, or from your car or the bus to the office, the store, the post office, the gym, anywhere? Do you walk, hike, jog, bike, or camp on weekends? What about going to flea markets, farmers' markets, lawn sales? Do you run out to get the newspaper from the front step, maybe the mail from your mailbox? Do you take advantage of the first warm weekend of the year to have coffee at an outdoor café? Do you hang your wash outside? Stand in line for a Saturday matinee movie? Sit in the yard chatting with your neighbor? Wait for your child outside the school door? Walk your dog?

The less you protect yourself outdoors, the greater your risk for wrinkles and other signs of skin aging, and even eye damage.

TIP FROM DR. COURTIN

To keep sun off your face, make sure the brim of your visor, cap, or hat is at least three inches long. Wear proper clothing, too. UV rays can easily penetrate the average T-shirt.

MYTH: I certainly don't need sun protection today—the sun's not even out.

While UV radiation can be blocked by dark, thick clouds, it readily penetrates clouds that are thin or fluffy. Although you might not actually see the sun high in the sky on a hazy day, its dangerous UV rays are reaching you as if it were shining brightly. In fact, by reflecting and refracting the sun's rays back to the surface of the earth, some clouds may even be responsible for amplifying UV radiation.

MYTH: My best friend uses a great sun-protection cream and never burns. I'll just use the same thing and I'll be fine!

No two women, no two skin types, are the same—and nowhere is this more evident than in reaction to sun exposure! Chances are that your girl-friend's skin type is sufficiently different from yours that not only shouldn't you be using the cream she uses, but also you each should be using sun-protection cream—as well as other skin-care products—custom-designed according to the numerous factors that make each of you who you are.

Fitzpatrick Classification for Skin Types and Reaction to Sun

Skin Type	Color	Reaction to UVA	Reaction to Sun
Type I	Caucasian; blond or red hair, freckles, fair skin, blue eyes	Very Sensitive	Always burns easily, never tans; very fair skin tone
Type II	Caucasian; blond or red hair, freckles, fair skin, blue eyes or green eyes	Very Sensitive	Usually burns easily, tans with difficulty; fair skin tone
Type III	Darker Caucasian, light Asian	Sensitive	Burns moderately, tans gradually; fair to medium skin tone
Type IV	Mediterranean, Asian, Hispanic	Moderately Sensitive	Rarely burns, always tans well; medium skin tone
Type V	Middle Eastern, Latin, light-skinned black, Indian	Minimally Sensitive	Very rarely burns, tans very easily; olive or dark skin tone
Type VI	Dark-skinned black	Least Sensitive	Never burns, deeply pigmented; very dark skin tone

In 1975, Thomas B. Fitzpatrick, MD, PhD, of Harvard Medical School, developed a classification system for skin typing. This system was based on a person's complexion and responses to sun exposure.

Make Exposure to the Sun Safer

Timing

If you insist on getting a tan, at least go about it in a wise, gradual way. Since skin newly exposed to the sun—especially when the sun is at its strongest—is at greatest risk for damage, plan your exposure according to a logical schedule. Sunbathe when the sun it not at its peak. The sun's hottest hours are between 10:00 A.M. and 2:00 P.M. (11:00 and 3:00 during daylight saving time). Start tanning before summer sets in, and incrementally increase session time, but never stay out longer than fifteen or twenty minutes at a time. With this approach, as you enter periods when the sun is most intense, your skin will have its initial tan to partially protect you while your color deepens. Still, always use sun-protection cream.

Use Sunscreen Properly

Whenever you are going to be in the sun, always use a sunblock cream with an SPF (sun-protection factor) of 15 or higher. If you are fair-skinned, choose an SPF of 30. Ideally, the cream should be applied fifteen to thirty minutes before you go outdoors. How much should you use? A good rule of thumb is to use the equivalent of a shot glass full of sunscreen.

Make sure you cover all areas of your body that will be exposed to the sun. Do an inventory, asking yourself, "If they're going to be exposed, have I covered my arms, back, chest, face, feet, hands, legs, neck, and stomach? What about my not-so-obvious places like armpits, earlobes, soles of feet, backs of knees, and scalp?" And don't be stingy with your sun-protection cream! You may not be applying enough for adequate coverage.

Reapply sunscreen at least every two hours. According to studies, if you wait more than two and a half hours, you're five times more likely to get burned than if you follow the two-hour rule. If you are playing sports, reapply every hour: Your cream rinses off with perspiration and rubs off at contact with other people and the ground. If you go into the water, reapply your cream as soon as you come out.

Wear Proper Clothing

When you go outside, wear a hat with a brim or visor that measures three inches or more. Try to expose as little of your skin as possible by wearing proper clothing. Note that T-shirts are not adequate protection from the sun; UV rays go right through the average T-shirt. Ideally, you should wear a garment to cover your thighs. If your clothing becomes wet, change it. The UV-protection power of wet garments can be cut in half. And don't forget your sunglasses. They should be 100 percent UV-blocking. Wraparound sunglasses protect you best, as they shade the sides of your face and of your eyes.

As recommended in the previous chapter, a balanced, varied diet especially rich in antioxidant vegetables and fruit is your ironclad defense against the accumulation of free radicals. Think of good nutrition as "internal sun-protection."

In addition to using a good sunblock and eating a balanced diet, to make sure you are doing all you can to prevent the negative and enhance the positive of sun exposure is it important to use customized skin-care products that clean and protect your skin: cleansers, toners, masks, moisturizers, and special formulas designed for the sensitive area around your eyes.

We Need *Some* Sunshine

After all these warnings about exposure to the sun, it may sound contradictory, but we all need some sunlight. The sun is not your enemy; only the abuse of it is. In fact, the sun actually plays some vital roles—such as being part of the metabolic and chemical processes that produce your body's vitamin D, especially important for bone health. And within the past two decades, attention has been focused on Seasonal Affective Disorder (SAD), characterized by incidents of depression during the winter months and alleviated—often completely—once spring and summer sunlight returns. It's important to strike a balance between being sun-phobic and sun-obsessed.

chapter 7

Key Five:

Recognize the Benefits of Exercise

THERE'S MORE GOOD NEWS ABOUT EXERCISE: It is excellent for your skin! Like proper nutrition, exercise benefits your entire body—inside and out, including your skin. Exercise gives you that natural, radiant look of health. It's the kind of look that cannot be replicated by artificial means, the look that leaps out at you from the covers of fitness magazines—featuring people who look like they just got off a surfboard or out of an aerobics class! Although we can't all resemble magazine models, we can unquestionably have one thing in common with them: the appearance of physical and emotional vitality that comes from getting your limbs moving, your heart pumping, your blood flowing, and your cells oxygenated.

Make Time for Exercise

Entire books—entire careers—have been devoted to enumerating the benefits of exercise, overall and for specific body parts and systems. The following brief list is intended to inspire the most inveterate sofa-sitter to lace up those sneakers. Exercise will:

- ❧ Boost circulation. Better blood flow increases oxygen and nutrient supply to every cell of your body and helps ensure efficient transport of waste products from your cells. This cleanses and nourishes your skin from within, contributing to a bright, younger-looking complexion.

- ❧ Aid in the healthful development of collagen. Collagen makes up 75 percent of your skin and helps it stay firm.

- ❧ Induce restful sleep, offering your skin added opportunities to revitalize and fewer opportunities to suffer the bags, dark circles, and drabness that follow sleepless nights. (It also reduces grumpiness—which causes scowl lines on your face.) People are usually so focused on the effort exercise demands that they don't realize good sleep is a benefit.

- ❧ Speed your metabolism. Faster metabolism means faster calorie-burning, which means less fat stored in your body.

- Keep your gastrointestinal track working like a well-oiled machine, helping you steer clear of constipation and the sallow skin tone that often accompanies it.

- Accelerate the activity of your endocrine glands, responsible for coordinating the functions that keep your system in balance.

- Fire up your immune system, which protects you from disease and infection. Former cancer patients often attribute their remission and recovery to the fact that they were extremely disciplined about exercising before the onset of their illnesses.

- Strengthen bones and muscles if training is moderate. Intense training—especially in heat and humidity—can do just the opposite, as calcium is lost with perspiration. Increasing calcium intake helps here. It is not true that aging invariably means developing fragile bones and weak muscles. Nothing could be further from the truth if strength training is part of your fitness regimen. Also called resistance training, strength training involves performing a series of movements against resistance, such as resistance bands or handheld weight bars. Resistance training also burns fat and increases stamina.

- Tone skin during and after significant weight loss and after pregnancy. Losing weight if you need to is great, but if you've slimmed down from a large size, your skin won't just naturally spring back from its previous stretched-out state. Without doing specific toning exercises and getting good overall workouts, you'll have sagging and bagging skin to deal with.

❧ Release endorphins. Naturally generated in the brain, endorphins are internal pain-killers produced by the body. When endorphins are released into our bloodstream, our pain perception diminishes, as does our perceived—and often real—level of stress. The amount released during a vigorous workout—especially intensive, repetitive activities such as running, biking, rowing, or stair-climbing—triggers a sense of physical and emotional well-being. Paradoxically, an endorphin release can make you feel both relaxed and energized.

Linked to the brain's "pleasure center," endorphins can increase self-esteem, reduce depression and anxiety, and generally put you in a good mood during and immediately following your workout. Some people feel great for the entire rest of the day. One of my favorite exercise stories is about a friend who is very short and skinny—and a dedicated amateur cyclist. His job frequently requires him to attend meetings with daunting superstars of his industry, most of whom are at least a head taller, much bulkier, and several professional ranks higher than he is. Whenever I ask him if he feels intimidated in the conference room, he looks at me as if I've just landed from another planet. "Me? Intimidated? Not possible!" he always answers. "I just make sure I bike a couple of dozen extra miles on those mornings. No one and nothing can touch me after that!"

A popular French word for "nervous, tense, on edge" is *crispé*. If you think that looks like "crispy," you're right. Synonyms for "crispy" are "brittle," "crunchy," "crusty," and "hard." Now, you wouldn't want your face and neck to look like that, would you? Of course not! This is why invigorating, endorphin-producing, stress-busting exercise must be part of your regimen for beautiful skin and overall health.

Unfortunately, we all don't have my friend's luxury of being able to start our days on the bike trail—or on the running path, in the swimming pool, at the gym, or even in our living rooms with a workout video and a mat. But the excuse of lack of time for exercise is just that: an excuse. The longer you go without regular exercise, the harder it will be to stay in good health.

Take an Activity Inventory

If you say you would love to exercise but just don't have—or can't find—the time, try the following. During the period from Sunday morning to Saturday night of a given week, carry a notebook with you, and write down as many of your activities as possible, including all television programs watched. Include every routine activity such as brushing your teeth, making morning coffee, and putting away your clothes at night. Include every unexpected activity such as having a leaky faucet fixed, answering e-mail from your long-lost cousin, or making dinner for a sick friend. Next to each entry, note the amount of time it took. In addition, for each day, record the time you got up, the time you went to bed, and the hours and length of all meals, including snacks.

Once the week and your list are finished, take two highlighter pens of different colors. With one pen, mark those nonessential activities that you could have done without, or that were time fillers (leafing through a magazine, for instance, until dinner finished cooking). With the other pen, mark your television-watching times.

Then immediately put the list away for two weeks—during that time, do not touch it at all. When you go back and look at it, read it as if it were someone else's list. Keep in mind that the person who wrote this list has said that her schedule is so packed that she could not fit exercise into her day.

What will probably jump out at you is the number of hours spent doing…well…not too terribly much—even for someone who conceives of her life as one enormous, impenetrable block of obligation-laden drudgery. Adding up—and consolidating, if possible—all those "empty" minutes is sure to produce at least the amount of time needed for a nice daily walk around the block. You might even find yourself saying something like, "It's amazing that there was enough time for *that*…and *that*…and *that* but not for doing some sit-ups!"

Next, look at every activity—essential and nonessential alike—and ask yourself, "Could I have shaved any minutes off the time it took me to do this? If so, how many?" Did you, for instance, leave too early for your dental appointment—knowing you'd have time to kill on the other end—because you were bored sitting around the house? Did you take the long way home from work for no particular reason? In answering e-mail did you go into screens and screens of detail that wasn't asked for and that probably didn't get read? Write the number of "shaveable" minutes next to each activity and add them up. Then ask yourself if the world would come to an end if you went to bed fifteen or thirty minutes earlier most nights. If you did so, you could get up that much earlier and use this "found" time, when you're refreshed and energetic after a good night's sleep, to better advantage.

Finally, consider the amount of time spent with the culprit that might be single-handedly responsible for delaying your dose of endorphins: the television. This is a double offender if there ever was one. It's unfortunate enough that your television is stealing precious hours that could be devoted to exercise, but also it has been said that only a sleeping baby burns fewer calories than someone sitting still watching the tube.

The point is: Somewhere in that list of activities is an exercise schedule waiting to happen. However, if even this method does not help you find the time needed to set your body in motion, you *still* have no excuse. When you can't go to the gym, bring the gym to you, by making your entire world your workout space, and your daily activities your exercise routine. The following suggestions can get you started.

- *Never—that's* never—*take an elevator or escalator when you can use the stairs.* In very tall buildings, at least take the stairs *part of* the way up and down. You'll get a great mini-cardiovascular workout.

- *Walk to work.* If walking is not possible, then bike, jog, or roller-blade. If even *that* is not possible, then walk to the bus, subway, or train, get off one or more stops away from work, and walk the rest of the way. Leaving your car at home also means you're not adding more toxic pollutants to the air. At the very least, when you drive to work, park as far from the building as you can and walk the distance to the door. Reverse the process for the trip home and replicate it for every one your destinations.

- *Carry your own packages.* From the store to your car. From the car to your house. Ideally—if possible—from the store to your house. If this entails several trips, your cardiovascular system and muscles will be all the stronger for it.

- *Turn your lunch hour into an exercise break.* Walk around the building, campus, or block after eating a sandwich at your desk. If you're eating out, walk to and from the restaurant. Doing your errands on foot is another good way to build exercise into your lunch hour.

🐦 *Turn your break into an exercise break*. Take a short walk during your break.

🐦 *Seize every opportunity to do "invisible" exercises.* These exercises firm your muscles and help get rid of fatty tissue. Do them by tensing your abdomen, buttocks, hips, thighs, calves, or upper arms for five or six seconds, then releasing; rolling up onto your tiptoes, stretching out your calf muscles, rolling back down; curling in your toes, stretching your foot and shin muscles, uncurling and stretching your toes. While sitting straight in your chair at your desk, bring your shoulder blades as close together as possible, hold for a few seconds, release; press your feet hard into the floor for ten seconds, release; push onto the seat with your hands, try to raise yourself for several seconds, release. Do six to ten repetitions of each in one session. These and similar movements can be done discreetly in many surprising places—at the bus stop, on the bus, at your desk, waiting in line, even during meetings.

🐦 *Play with your kids—throw a ball, have a game of tag, roll in the grass together.* Bonuses include enjoying family time, helping your kids stay in shape, setting a good fitness example.

- *Laugh.* It's good for your stomach muscles, lungs, heart, head, and the people around you.

- *Turn off the television.* Walk over to do it—don't use the remote control! In fact, if you "have to" watch television, *never* use the remote control. Pretend it doesn't exist. Pretend it's broken. Pretend it never was invented. Get rid of it. Stand up and go over to the television to change the channels. If you're a machine-gun-speed channel surfer, so much the better! Stand up and go over every time. Ultimately, you'll give up and spend those precious minutes doing "real" exercise, or you'll reconcile yourself to the fact that you've turned your living room into a walking track.

Don't Overlook Skin Care When You Exercise

Don't forget skincare as part of your work out. With all the good intentions in the world, many women make a number of mistakes related to their skin care before, during, and after they exercise. The most blatant of these is neglecting their skin altogether.

Skin care should not be regarded as a chore or as an isolated activity but as a lifestyle. As we have seen regarding mental attitude, nutrition, exercise, and health in general, when you take care of your mind and body—every day in every way—your skin comes out a winner. And vice versa. Putting skin care on hold between the time you get up and the time you come in from running, for instance—or not protecting yourself from the elements while you're out there pounding the pavement because you're too busy worrying about keeping your heart rate up—is like putting breathing on hold while you're cooking: These are not, and thus should not be considered, mutually exclusive acts.

TIP FROM DR. COURTIN

No matter how late it is, no matter how tired you are after exercise, always cleanse, tone, and moisturize your skin before going to sleep. If not, you will pay for it in old-looking skin later on.

Remember the following tips to make sure your exercise program benefits your skin to the maximum:

- *Cleanse, tone, and moisturize your face and neck daily.* Do it when you get out of bed every day—whether you're starting that day with an exercise session or not. Not taking a shower until after your morning workout is understandable; not performing at least your basic morning skin-care ritual is abusive to your skin.

🐦 *Before you exercise, remove your makeup base, blush, face powder, and eye shadow.* If you don't do so, your perspiration will mix with these cosmetics, clogging your pores, and making one big mess of your skin. This step is especially important when you won't be able to wash your face immediately after working out. If you wouldn't be caught dead leaving the house without a trace of makeup, stick with just eyebrow pencil, mascara, and lipstick for your workouts.

🐦 *When exercising outdoors—summer or winter—make sure you're properly protected.* As mentioned earlier, use a sunscreen with an SPF of 15 or higher on all exposed areas, and reapply it every two hours. Wear a cap or visor with at least a three-inch brim and 100 percent UV-blocking, wraparound sunglasses. In summer, work out in loose-fitting, light-colored clothing that leaves as little skin exposed to the sun as comfortably possible. In winter, ward off chapped lips and skin with lip balm and an extra layer of moisturizer—both with built-in sun protection.

🐦 *Avoid snug clothing.* Super-snug spandex and nylon might dazzle them at the gym but these fabrics prevent air from reaching your skin and evaporating perspiration. With sweat now clogging your pores, those little red bumps commonly known as heat rash begin to form. Do not smother your skin! Let it breathe in garments of natural fibers such as cotton in the summer or, better yet, all year round in clothing specially made to wick moisture away from your body as you exercise; it's available at sporting goods stores.

- *Prevent chafing.* Spread petroleum jelly on body parts likely to rub against each other or clothing (thigh against thigh, nipple against workout bra, underarms). Never put petroleum jelly on your face—it clogs your pores.

- *Do not put dirty equipment next to your skin.* Before slipping on gear such as helmets and protective padding, clean it to the greatest extent possible. Why host someone else's germs and sweat or even your own if you can avoid it?

- *Stay well hydrated.* Dehydration is harmful to your body and your skin. Do not depend on your body's thirst mechanism to tell you when to drink. Chances are, it's not as reliable as you think. Drink eight ounces of water even before starting your workout. During your workout, drink eight ounces of water every fifteen to twenty minutes; if this presents a problem, aim for every half hour and never go longer than an hour of exercise without drinking that amount. Drink eight to ten ounces right after your workout; at this point fruit juices are also okay, but they might cause gastrointestinal discomfort during exertion.

If you want to try a sports drink, avoid gastrointestinal problems by getting used to it gradually, sipping it in progressively greater quantities during each workout while rounding out your fluid intake with water. Stay away from carbonated drinks during exertion—all those bubbles bouncing around in your stomach can upset it.

chapter 8

Key Six:

Get Your Skin a Personal Trainer!

SOME IDEAS SEEM BOTH SIMPLE AND REVOLUTIONARY at the same time—the ideas that make us slap our palms against our foreheads and declare, "Now, why didn't *I* think of that?"

One of the clearest examples of this is the use of skin-care products specially conceived and formulated to meet each woman's unique skin-care needs. Think of these customized skin-care products as a "personal trainer for your skin." Within the past twenty years, much progress has been made both in the scientific study of skin and in the development of beauty treatments. Because we have come to know more and more about why and how skin ages and reacts to external elements, we are better equipped to create customized products for keeping it healthy, young-looking, and beautiful.

As awesome as Mother Nature is, she alone is not enough in caring for your skin: It needs to be nurtured with customized—personalized—products that can help you maximize the positives with which nature endows it, and minimize the negatives with which she confronts it.

If you lived in an "ideal" world, the resources and tools that nature has given you would be almost enough for surviving and thriving, for being and remaining as healthy, fit, and beautiful as possible. In some remote areas of the world, these resources and tools are in fact almost enough: areas without pollution, without stress, without junk food, without—in some cases—even a word in the local language for "war"!

But, as you will see in this chapter, the vital word here is "almost," since even in the most pristine, idyllic settings, a woman's skin is programmed to age and to react to the many changes that her body—and mind—experience over the course of her lifetime.

The next best thing to an ideal world is one in which help—nurturing—from "the outside" is available. Even better is one in which help is *personalized* to meet your individual, distinct needs as you face the challenges that less-than-ideal biological, emotional, and environmental realities ceaselessly and relentlessly throw your way.

The notion of personal trainers is not new. But while hiring personal trainers was once reserved for movie stars, now such training is available to the general public. If you go to a gym, you already know that personal trainers are readily available to help you make the most of your workout sessions.

The concept of made-to-order personal-care products—"personal trainers" for your skin—goes far back in history. Perfumes and cosmetics were specially blended for empresses. Remedies for all sorts of illnesses and conditions were concocted for Roman senators, medieval abbots, Renaissance princesses, generals, Industrial Age entrepreneurs. Indeed, in the days before the Internet, the shopping mall, and even the local pharmacy, the only way to obtain such products was, if you were poor, to make them yourself from trusted family recipes. If you were rich, you could have them made for you by alchemists and chemists, physicians, and private parfumeurs.

In some areas of the world even now, local healers spend their days and nights caring for members of tribes and communities with custom-designed potions and care routines.

What is new is the notion that every woman deserves—and can have access to—attention that used to be reserved for the very rich, famous, and powerful or for individuals in extremely isolated areas of the globe.

So just what are the similarities between a personal trainer for your body and a personal trainer for your skin? These can be summed up with the acronym A.P.P.E.A.L., which stands for **A**ssess, **P**ersonalize, **P**amper, **E**ncourage, **A**im, and **L**ead.

Assessing Your Needs

For your body: A good personal trainer assesses your workout needs according to your state of health and fitness, your goals, your capabilities, and lifestyle details such as your eating and sleeping patterns, levels of stress, available time, and more.

For your skin: The vital role of an in-store skin-care consultant cannot be overstated. She is there for you. She listens to you and answers your questions. She assesses and continually monitors the specific, distinct needs of your skin and suggests how your personal trainer—your customized skin-care regimen—can meet your specific needs.

TIP FROM DR. COURTIN

Always use products adapted to your own, personal skin-care needs. Your twice-daily, morning and night, cleansing routine is crucial to the health and beauty of your skin.

Personalizing Care

For your body: According to the assessment results, the consultant custom designs and updates your fitness plan.

For your skin: Customization is the bedrock of personalized skin care. It is the keystone of the ideal skin-care products and the foundation upon which a skin-care consultant bases her recommendations. Customized care must concentrate on a woman's continually changing needs throughout her lifetime. Using the same cream to care for each woman's complexly unique skin type and conditions through her entire life would be like buying the same dress in the same size and the same color for every woman in the country and asking that they never take it off.

Pampering Yourself

For your body: In addition to communicating facts and figures, instructions, and suggestions, a good personal trainer makes sure you feel like the center of the universe: cared for, supported in your efforts, understood, and, yes, pampered. Far from representing a public-relations "technique," this has a very concrete, sensible rationale: Being pampered makes you feel better. When you feel better, you're more relaxed. When you're more relaxed, those facts, figures, instructions, and suggestions—even if unfamiliar and daunting—are more easily accepted, absorbed, and implemented. You progress faster and attain your goals with greater ease.

For your skin: The effects of pampering are similar when it comes to skin care. In study after study, and through enough anecdotal evidence to fill shelves' worth of books, it has been shown that something as seemingly insignificant as the cool, smooth feel of a face cream, the fresh fragrance of a sunblock, or the purchase of a single lipstick in the season's latest color, helps you feel happy, optimistic, confident, and pampered. Personalizing your skin care puts you truly at the center, focusing on you, on the internal and external influences that make your skin unique, and on meeting those unique skin-care needs.

Encouragement

For your body: A good personal trainer knows that it is essential to encourage you. She knows that encouragement inspires you to press further and further toward your goals. The trainer knows when to encourage you most, noticing your subtle signals when you need an extra little push.

For your skin: When our world makes too many demands on us it is difficult to find the motivation, energy, or time to give our skin all the attention it needs. But the greatest encouragement of all comes from positive results: Good skin care is its own built-in cheering section.

Aim for Good Results

For your body: A good personal trainer helps you set and continuously review and revise your individualized exercise goals, as well as evaluate your progress toward attaining them. The trainer knows that aims must be measurable and reasonable: If they are set too high, you will feel defeated and discouraged; too low, and you will under perform.

For your skin: An expert skin-care consultant follows your skin's evolution through all its phases. She makes sure that your products are best suited to your individual requirements at all times under all circumstances. She continuously monitors and measures your progress toward optimal skin-care results.

Leading You in the Right Direction

For your body: Aware that fitness is a matter of overall health, a good personal trainer does more than merely assign a few series of sit-ups. The trainer takes the lead in helping you manage the wide range of factors that affect your whole person, integrating relevant advice into a comprehensive well-being plan.

For your skin: What is good for your skin is good for your entire body. The converse of this is true as well. Caring for your skin means learning about your biological phases and their effects; optimizing your mental attitude and emotional well-being; paying attention to your diet and good nutrition; keeping your system in top shape through regular exercise; limiting your exposure to elements such as wind, sun, extreme cold, and pollution; minimizing your levels of stress; ensuring proper amounts of sleep; and using skin-care products suited to your unique needs. Personalized skin care takes the lead as you pull all these challenging tasks together to achieve the results you want.

Conclusion

IF SOMEONE WOKE ME UP ABRUPTLY in the middle of the night and asked, "Quick! What is your one most important piece of advice about skin care?" there would not be a second's hesitation. My answer would be: Never forget that skin is an organ.

And, more fascinating than that, it is the *only* organ that you can treat directly. Of course, indirect skin-care "treatments" abound—and they have, to a great extent, been the subjects of this book: having a positive attitude, ensuring excellent nutrition, getting regular exercise, reducing stress, trying to avoid unsafe environmental conditions, paying special attention to the harmful effects of too much sun. All these contribute to the enduring health and beauty of your skin since, as I have said, what is good for your other organs is good for your skin, and vice versa.

But how fortunate that, where this organ is concerned, you can also add the direct touch—literally "touch"—by applying creams and lotions that properly protect, nourish, and nurture it! Now there are personalized products custom-made and adapted to answer your skin's individual and continually evolving needs throughout your lifetime.

Then I would pose a question to the person who had awakened me: "Why not take fullest advantage of everything available to care for your skin—indirectly and directly?" The solutions seem so easy. If you cut an apple in two and leave one half in the open air, it turns brown, spotty, old-looking, dry; but put the other half in lemon juice and it stays fresh-looking, bright, attractive, moist. The "lemon juice" your skin needs to keep it healthy and bright is a line of custom-designed skin products. Easy solutions, radiant results.

And all this at any age.

I like to compare the skin to machines in a factory. When you are twenty years old, the factory is new and its machines are well oiled and high-performing. Apart from regular maintenance, they don't demand too much attention. A decade or so down the line, the machines don't always function as before—but if you take special measures to keep them in top working order, your efforts usually pay off.

We have spoken about the beneficial use of plant extracts in skin-care products, and we extol the bountiful virtues and sing the well-deserved praises of plants as nature's personal-care gifts to us. But we also acknowledge that although these plant extracts may be 100 percent natural, it is utopian to think this means they are 100 percent efficient, effective, and safe. Therefore we utilize today's scientific resources, equipment, knowledge, and expertise to maximize plants' tremendous qualities and potential, resulting in the best skin-care products possible. How? Here are just a few of many examples:

- Science helps us extract from plants just the right elements for the desired product effect, be it cleansing, toning, moisturizing, soothing, exfoliating, or firming.

- Science allows us to stabilize the mixtures' various molecules, both natural and human-made, so that they do not interfere with each other's hard work, and so that they can each do their best job.

- Science permits the ingredients' molecules to increase the effect of or act synergistically with each other.

- Science ensures that products stay fresh and safe as you transport, use, and store them.

Starting with a "raw botanical" and creating a product that helps keep your skin healthy and beautiful, smells wonderful, and ensures easy and safe use demonstrates the important and fascinating synergy between science and nature.

At the very beginning of this book, I invited you to listen to your skin, to hear it tell you what it needs at all moments, in all situations. I asked that you give it the personalized attention and care that it—and you—deserve. I repeat that invitation, now more than ever. And now, as we say in French, "au revoir," or "See you later."

My Blend

AS YOU HAVE SEEN throughout this book, the story of a woman's biological and emotional life can be read on her skin. Both nature and nurture play a role. Nature involves such things as hormonal changes, pregnancy and childbirth, pre-menopause and menopause, and environmental assaults from sun, wind, and extreme temperatures. Your skin is also affected by your physiological and emotional reactions to life's daily stresses and by your nutrition and exercise habits. Nurture, or how you take care of you skin, is an equally important factor in the appearance of your skin.

In this framework, it is with pleasure that I present *My Blend*, the first line of highly personalized skin care in the cosmetics field.

The Philosophy behind *My Blend*

My Blend is a completely new approach to skin care and defines a new generation of "intelligent" skin care for life's various stages. It treats a woman's skin according to her individual evolving needs. This approach goes far beyond the market's conventional skin-care product categories that are usually recommended by skin type and age. It offers customized, extremely fine-tuned formulas built on a platform of scientific technology and completed with powerful bio-botanicals.

Young skin can look like old skin if not properly cared for, diminishing the significance of your chronological age. Further, the various reasons why your skin is oily, dry, or a combination are vastly more important than the occurrence of these conditions. So it seems unimaginable that a single, one-size-fits-all product labeled, for example, "for oily skin" is the best product for your skin. Nor can a single product address the needs of all women under various biological, emotional, and environmental circumstances—conditions that are potential threats to your skin's health and beauty.

The first and foremost mission of the entire *My Blend* line is to protect and stimulate your skin's natural defense systems. How does this work? The exclusive patented complex called "CellSynergy" is the scientific core of all *My Blend* products. This biotechnical complex is able to fight the effects of stress well before it can have any impact on the skin, protecting and preserving skin's structures, and fortifying it day after day. Thus, extremely well defended, your skin will be stronger and healthier, better able to face external and internal aggressors, as well as the general aging process. CellSynergy's benefits are multifold:

- It protects Langerhans cells, the active line of immunity defense inside your skin, and one of the most important systems in your body for fighting oxidative stress, pollution damage, infections, and so forth. As you age, your Langerhans cells weaken and their number diminishes.

- It protects the skin's nerve endings. Through close interaction with your skin's cells, your nervous system can modulate or control all of your skin's functions, including substance synthesis, moisturizing, immunity, and cellular differentiation or proliferation. Nerve cells have a low renewal potential, and are modified with age.

- It supplies your skin with crucially needed antioxidants for protection against damaging free radicals.

Getting Started with *My Blend*

At the *My Blend* counter, in department stores, you will first have a detailed analysis performed by a highly trained skin-care consultant. This expert will take into account your specific needs and help you to select the particular Essential Formula (out of the eight existing) that is best for your present skin condition. If there is a special temporary skin problem or urgency, she will propose that you include the second level of personalization: a "megadose" of well-targeted and super-concentrated "Actives" injected into your Essential Formula for an "emergency" treatment. This pre-measured dose of special ingredients exists in five different formulas and comes in small glass syringes called Emergency Boosters. (Note that the glass syringes, which contain no needles, are used only to inject the formula into a jar of cream.)

The skin consultant will assess the many factors that can influence your skin's health, for example, if you are:

- In your twenties, pregnant, stressed by overwork, living in a pollution-saturated city, plagued by dry skin, or spending too much time in the sun.

- A woman of forty, who is going through pre-menopause and has oily skin and a tendency to indulge in fast food.

- Running marathons at age fifty, eating well, and taking excellent care of yourself in general and of your skin in particular.

- In your sixties and convinced, after a lifetime of feeling unattractive, that by this age nothing will help you look and feel your best.

My Blend Products

My Blend introduces the era of "adjustable skin care," in which the skin-care products for your regimen are perfectly fine-tuned for your skin—just like a custom-made garment. The products you take home represent one of the 225 possible blending combinations between the Essential Formula family (Day & Night, lotions and creams) and the Booster family. The third product family is composed of "Specifics." This includes two eye creams, a skin brightener, a daily sun protector, smart rinse-off cleansers, and a very efficient acne treatment fluid.

The Essential Formula range is organized by colors and by numbers, from 01 to 08. Each formula jar/bottle has been assigned a specific color. The creams come in large sizes for your daily needs. Each formula contains the exact quantity of "CellSynergy" adapted to the skin condition it is meant to treat, as well as a number of powerful bio-botanicals targeted for your specific skin needs. The Essential Formulas are extremely fine-tuned and concentrated products designed for individual and evolving needs during every life stage. They are complete treatments that cover absolutely all your "normal" day and night skin needs. But emergencies happen, and when they do, Boosters allow you to take personalization to the next level. Use your Mini-Lab (a smaller size of your cream or lotion formula), choose the Booster your skin needs, and inject the premeasured dose. Blend thoroughly and enjoy this immediate power surge on your skin. According to the program determined with your *My Blend* skin-care expert, you will open one or two color-coded Booster syringes and blend either the complete contents of one Booster into one Mini-Lab cream/lotion size, or one half of each of them into the Day Formula and the other two halves into the Night Formula. The boosted formula represents a two-week cure treatment.

Keep these points in mind:

- Since your skin can absorb only so many elements at any given time, it is advisable to create your weekly batch of cream using no more than two types of Boosters. Should your skin-care consultant suggest that you need more than two types of Boosters, you can alternate, using one or two types one week and one or two different types the next.

- Since the Boosters' ingredients are most effective the fresher they are, it is advisable to mix a cream-Booster batch just ample enough for one week's application and to do so right before you are about to start using the batch (Sunday night or Monday morning, for instance, if your "batch week" begins on Monday).

- Because both the Essentials Formulas creams/lotions and the Boosters come from the *My Blend* laboratories, their compatibility and synergy are ensured.

A Mini-Chemistry Lesson

As you can imagine, detailing the diverse properties of all the ingredients—as well as the work they perform—would fill countless chapters and remind some of us of those long hours spent in chemistry and biology class. But the "little chemist" you met in the introduction to this book cannot resist sharing at least a bit of his lifelong passion for any substance that enhances the health and beauty of a woman's skin.

Each of the numerous *My Blend* ingredients, be they plant-extract-based or biotechnical, has a story to tell. Some of those stories—in the case of the bio-botanicals—go back literally thousands of years. Some of the biotechnicals echo countless dedicated hours spent in a laboratory by tireless scientists in search of that perfect result.

In the text that follows, I will discuss several samples—first, three biotechnicals and then, three botanicals. All of them have been chosen for *My Blend* because they are the most active, high-performing substances possible for the jobs we are asking them to do.

- Thymulen: This synthetic ingredient created from the most recent biotechnical research programs offers an advanced immune protection shield to the skin's natural defense systems. It helps protect the Langerhans cells, maintaining your skin's self-defense capacity while encouraging its renewal capabilities. As a part of the "CellSynergy" complex, it is used in all eight Essential Formulas, with an increasing level through the range. Skin becomes healthier and more radiant.

- Glistin: This biotechnical ingredient is a neuro protector and regenerator. Part of the "CellSynergy" Day Complex, it helps preserve your skin's nerve endings, maintaining and stimulating all skin functions, encouraging skin renewal throughout the day.

- Imudilin: Designed as a neuro-protection energizer, this biotechnical ingredient is part of the "CellSynergy" Night Complex. It works overnight to restore cellular immune defense, stimulate cellular metabolism, and repair cellular damage incurred during the day.

- Ginkgo biloba: A natural ingredient, it comes from an ancient species of tree; its leaves are rich in antioxidants, which block the formation of free radicals in the skin. This antioxidant also works to moisturize, tone, and restructure your skin cells. It is used in the Redness Rescue Booster.

❧ Ginseng: A plant from Asia, its root is called the "flower of life." The Chinese claim that its overall stimulating properties preserve youthfulness. Ginseng is an anti-free radical, containing many nutrients, especially vitamins. It works to stimulate, tone, and restructure your skin cells. Ginseng extract is used in the Speedy Recovery Booster.

❧ Aloe Vera: The sap from the leaves of this plant is rich in vitamins, enzymes, minerals, proteins, and amino acids and is used to hydrate, soothe, and protect your skin from environmental aggressions. Aloe vera was cherished by the ancient Egyptians, Romans, Greeks, Arabs, Indians, and Chinese. It has been used through the ages for cosmetic and curative purposes. Cleopatra is said to have attributed her beauty to aloe gel. Legend has it that Aristotle convinced Alexander the Great to capture the island of Socotra, rich with a supply of aloe, so his soldiers' wounds could be treated with the precious sap. Aloe vera is used in the Night Formula 08 (mature, postmenopausal skin).

My Blend Skin-Care Products

Day Formulas (6 Lotions/4 Creams) Face and Neck

01/ Oil Crisis Control Day & Night Lotion (refillable pump-bottle,
      50 and 15 ml)

02/ Calm & Controlled Day Lotion (refillable pump-bottle, 50 and 15 ml)

03/ Stress Management Day Lotion (refillable pump-bottle, 50 and 15 ml)

04/ Balance of Power Day Lotion (refillable pump-bottle, 50 and 15 ml)

05/ Early Age Alert Day Lotion (refillable pump-bottle, 50 and 15 ml)

05/ Early Age Alert Day Crème (refillable jar, 50 and 15 ml)

06/ Prescribed Comfort Day Lotion (refillable pump-bottle, 50 and 15 ml)

06/ Prescribed Comfort Day Crème (refillable jar, 50 and 15 ml)

07/ Change for the Better Day Crème (refillable jar, 50 and 15 ml)

08/ Potent Age Antidote Day Crème (refillable jar, 50 and 15 ml)

Night Formulas (7 Creams) Face and Neck

02/ Calm & Controlled Night Crème (refillable jar, 50 and 15 ml)

03/ Stress Management Night Crème (refillable jar, 50 and 15 ml)

04/ Balance of Power Night Crème (refillable jar, 50 and 15 ml)

05/ Early Age Alert Night Crème (refillable jar, 50 and 15 ml)

06/ Prescribed Comfort Night Crème (refillable jar, 50 and 15 ml)

07/ Change for the Better Night Crème (refillable jar, 50 and 15 ml)

08/ Potent Age Antidote Night Crème (refillable jar, 50 and 15 ml)

THE COURTIN CONCEPT

Emergency Boosters

Speedy Recovery (glass syringe, 1.5 ml)

Redness Rescue (glass syringe, 1.5 ml)

Moisture Immersion (glass syringe, 1.5 ml)

Radiant Burst (glass syringe, 1.5 ml)

Antioxidant Surge (glass syringe, 1.5 ml)

Specifics

Accelerated Acne Antidote (bottle, 50 ml)

Light & Luminous (bottle, 50 ml)

Power Veil SPF 40 (bottle, 50 ml)

Eye Creams

Time Resistant Eye Crème (jar, 15 ml)

Time Reversing Eye Crème (jar, 15 ml)

Cleansers

Caring Cream Cleanser (tube, 125 ml)

Detoxifying & Purifying Cleanser (tube, 125 ml)

Skin Polishing Cleanser (tube, 125 ml)

My Blend Questionnaire

By completing the following questionnaire and taking it to a *My Blend* consultant at a department store carrying the My Blend line, you will help the skin-care expert there to personalize your unique skin-care regimen.

1. Your age: _____

2. Your profession: _____

3. Number of children: _____

4. Are you: ☐ pregnant   ☐ premenopausal
             ☐ going through menopause   ☐ postmenopausal

5. Major illnesses, if any: _____

    _____

    _____

6. Cosmetic surgery, if any: _____

    _____

    _____

7. Types of injuries / scars, if any: _____

    _____

    _____

8. Do you live in :   ☐ a big city   ☐ a medium-size city
             ☐ a small town   ☐ a the countryside

9. How many hours/day are you in the sun:

   for daily activities _____ for leisure activities _____

10. Do you eat: ☐ healthfully ☐ moderately healthfully

    ☐ moderately unhealthfully ☐ unhealthfully?

11. Do you exercise (yes / no)? _____

    If yes, types and frequency of exercise: _____

    _____

    _____

    _____

12. Your life is: ☐ very stressful ☐ moderately stressful

    ☐ moderately unstressful ☐ unstressful

For more information, please visit

www.myblendbeauty.com

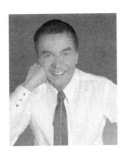

About the Author

I N T H E H E A L T H A N D B E A U T Y I N D U S T R Y , Dr. Olivier Courtin-Clarins is known as a "skin guru." Since 2000 he has been the managing director of the Clarins Group, maker of the Clarins line of cosmetics, the European leader in premium skin-care products, with products sold through a selective distribution network of 19,000 points of sale in more than 150 countries.

After studying medicine at the Faculty of Paris V-René Descartes, Dr. Courtin practiced as an orthopedic surgeon, as a specialist in treating sport accidents, and as an emergency specialist. He worked as senior registrar at Foch Hospital in Suresnes until he became Clarins's research manager in 1995 and later joined their board of directors.

Dr. Courtin-Clarins is President of both ARTHRITIS, the first French Foundation to help in the research against chronic inflammatory rheumatism, and the Supervisory Board of the company Mugler SA. He is also involved in presenting the Most Dynamisant Woman Award, an acknowledgment of women around the world who fund projects to help underprivileged children.

Dr. Courtin-Clarins is also a member of the Racing Club of France, an avid golfer, and a world traveler. He lives in Paris and has twin daughters.

He is the author of several works, published in France and abroad, on orthopedic surgery and dermatology.